LAB
RESULTS
MADE EASY

For Mum, Dad, Kamal
and Rizwan

LAB
RESULTS
MADE EASY

NAZIA HUSSAIN

MBBCh, DRCOG, DCH, DFSRH, PG Cert in Medical Education
General Practitioner, Aneurin Bevan University Health Board, NHS Wales

Consultant Editors:

NADIA EL-FARHAN
Consultant Clinical Biochemist, Aneurin Bevan University Health Board, NHS Wales

SARAH GODDARD
Consultant Clinical Immunologist, University Hospitals of North Midlands

CHRIS GREGORY
Consultant Haematologist, Royal Albert Edward Infirmary, Wrightington, Wigan and Leigh Teaching Hospitals NHS Foundation Trust

ELIZABETH KUBIAK
Consultant Microbiologist, Aneurin Bevan University Health Board, NHS Wales

SHALIKA PALANGASINGHE
Consultant Microbiologist, Aneurin Bevan University Health Board, NHS Wales

Scion

© Scion Publishing Limited, 2025

ISBN 9781914961601

A CIP catalogue record for this book is available from the British Library.

Scion Publishing Limited

The Old Hayloft, Vantage Business Park, Bloxham Road, Banbury OX16 9UX, UK

www.scionpublishing.com

Important Note from the Publisher
The information contained within this book was obtained by Scion Publishing Ltd from sources believed by us to be reliable. However, while every effort has been made to ensure its accuracy, no responsibility for loss or injury whatsoever occasioned to any person acting or refraining from action as a result of information contained herein can be accepted by the authors or publishers.

Readers are reminded that medicine is a constantly evolving science and while the authors and publishers have ensured that all dosages, applications and practices are based on current indications, there may be specific practices which differ between communities. You should always follow the guidelines laid down by the manufacturers of specific products and the relevant authorities in the country in which you are practising.

Although every effort has been made to ensure that all owners of copyright material have been acknowledged in this publication, we would be pleased to acknowledge in subsequent reprints or editions any omissions brought to our attention.

Registered names, trademarks, etc. used in this book, even when not marked as such, are not to be considered unprotected by law.

Typeset by Evolution Design & Digital Ltd (Kent)
Printed in the UK
Last digit is the print number: 10 9 8 7 6 5 4 3 2 1

Contents

Chapter 2: Haematology   115

ABNORMAL RESULTS

Part II: Requesting investigations

Chapter 6: Signs and symptoms   235

Preface

Back in 2000, *Lab Results Made Easy* was little more than a hopeful idea. As a GP navigating full, fast-paced days, I often found myself wasting valuable time hunting for guidance on how best to manage abnormal results. In moments of need, reliable answers were rarely at hand – often scattered across books/websites or designed primarily for secondary care.

Even amongst colleagues, there were clear variations in how we approached common abnormalities – for example, when to order an ECG for hypokalaemia or when an emergency admission was warranted.

I remember thinking: *What if there was a single, practical resource designed for GPs – something that could save time, reduce uncertainty, and build confidence in clinical decisions for better patient outcomes?* There had to be a better way than ad hoc searches or spending precious minutes calling specialists or on-call teams.

That idea gradually became a vision – the vision has only become a reality thanks to the incredible people who have supported me throughout this long journey.

Acknowledgements

First and foremost, all praise and thanks be to **Allah** for granting me the ability and opportunity to complete this work.

To my **family**, thank you for your unwavering support, love and prayers. Every one of my achievements stands upon your solid shoulders. **Mum** and **Dad**, you were especially patient during the long, long hours when I would disappear behind closed doors writing and refining flowcharts.

A heartfelt thanks to all those who contributed to reviewing the book, including **Kalpana Harris**, **Katerina Heydon** and **Ifeoma Ujomu**. A special thanks to the chapter editors who have been pivotal in providing specialist input and bridging the interface between primary and secondary care when managing abnormal tests. Thank you for your time, effort and unwavering commitment (in chapter order): **Nadia El-Farhan**, **Chris Gregory**, **Sarah Goddard**, **Elizabeth Kubiak** and **Shalika Palangasinghe**.

I am indebted to **Jonathan** and the amazing team at **Scion Publishing** for believing in my vision and transforming a distant hope into a printed reality. And **Clare**, thank you for your patience editing such a complicated and fiddly project.

Finally, my sincere hope is that *Lab Results Made Easy* not only supports better patient care and outcomes but also proves to be a practical, time-saving companion for my primary care colleagues – those who do extraordinary work every day with unwavering skill, dedication and resilience in often challenging circumstances.

"None of us is as smart as all of us."
— *Ken Blanchard*

About the author and editors

Nazia Hussain

Dr Nazia Hussain is a GP based in South Wales, UK. She has a special interest in women's health and is a headache specialist working for the 'National Migraine Centre' charity. With a keen interest in medical education, Nazia has previously been a Deputy Editor for *InnovAit*, the official journal of the Royal College of General Practitioners, and has contributed to the *Oxford Handbook of General Practice* (5th edition) as a guest author.

Nadia El-Farhan – editor of *Chapter 1*

Dr El-Farhan has run the Aneurin Bevan University Health Board's Lipid and Metabolic Kidney Stone services since 2012. She also runs a fortnightly Dynamic Function test clinic and the joint Paediatric Lipid Clinic. She is the Clinical Lead for Medical Biochemistry, Chair of the Point of Care Testing Committee and a tutor for the MSc in Preventative Cardiovascular Medicine at the University of South Wales. Dr El-Farhan's main clinical interests include cardiovascular risk management, familial hypercholesterolaemia, primary hypertriglyceridaemia, hypertriglyceridaemia-associated pancreatitis and kidney stone prevention. Her PhD thesis explored assay-specific cortisol cut-offs for the short Synacthen test, and she maintains a strong interest in cortisol measurement and evaluation of the hypothalamic–pituitary–adrenal axis. Other biochemical interests include calcium metabolism, hyponatraemia, hypomagnesaemia, refeeding syndrome and investigation of incongruous biochemical results.

Chris Gregory – editor of *Chapter 2*

In addition to his role as a Consultant Haematologist, Dr Gregory is also Clinical Director of Cancer Services at the Royal Albert Edward Infirmary, part of Wrightington, Wigan and Leigh Teaching Hospitals NHS Foundation Trust. He started work there as a Consultant Haematologist in November 2013 after completing training in the Merseyside region. He has a lead role in managing patients with lymphoma within the Trust and for overseeing the nurse-led anticoagulation clinics, and is also the Chair of the Thrombosis Committee.

Sarah Goddard – editor of *Chapter 3*

Sarah Goddard's areas of expertise are immunodeficiency, allergy and immunology laboratory services. Dr Goddard completed her undergraduate training in 1994 in Southampton. Since then she has worked in Stoke-on-Trent, Cambridge and Birmingham. It was during her PhD with the liver unit in Birmingham that she discovered her interest in immunology. She has been a consultant with University Hospitals of North Midlands since 2010 and during this time the allergy and laboratory service has been accredited and has achieved recognition as a specialist centre for allergy and immunodeficiency.

Elizabeth Kubiak – editor of *Chapter 4*

After qualifying in medicine from London University (Guy's and King's College Hospitals), Dr Kubiak trained in General Pathology and Microbiology in Bristol, further specialising in Medical Microbiology at St. George's Hospital, London and on the West Midlands Specialist Registrar rotation from Queen Elizabeth Hospital, Birmingham. Now semi-retired, Dr Kubiak has practised in the NHS as Consultant Medical Microbiologist to Aneurin Bevan Health Board in South Wales for over 30 years. She assisted on the Health Board's Research Scrutiny Committee for over 10 years, and was Health Board Infection Control Doctor for two terms of office. Dr Kubiak also served 12 years on the Veterinary Products Committee of DEFRA's Veterinary Medicines Department, and is still an active member of the All-Wales Microbiology Methods Development and Standardisation Group, and All-Wales Decontamination and Sterilisation Group. Dr Kubiak's special interests are antimicrobial stewardship, One Health / Zoonoses, and gastrointestinal infections.

Shalika Palangasinghe – editor of *Chapter 4*

Dr Shalika Palangasinghe completed her MBBS and postgraduate training in Medical Microbiology (Postgraduate Diploma and MD) in Sri Lanka and then joined Wythenshawe Hospital, Manchester as an honorary Specialist Registrar in Microbiology for one year. In 2017 she started her career as a Consultant Microbiologist in Sri Lanka. She worked as a Specialty Doctor in Microbiology at The Princess Alexandra NHS Trust, Harlow in 2020 and completed FRCPath in 2021. Dr Palangasinghe joined Aneurin Bevan University Health Board in South Wales in 2022 and is currently working as a Locum Consultant in Microbiology.

Abbreviations

AAT	alpha-1 antitrypsin	CVD	cardiovascular disease
ACEi	angiotensin-converting enzyme inhibitor	CXR	chest X-ray
		DCT	direct Coombs' test
ACR	albumin:creatinine ratio	DEXA	dual energy X-ray absorptiometry
ADH	antidiuretic hormone		
AKI	acute kidney injury	DGP	deamidated gliadin peptide
ALO	actinomyces-like organisms	DI	diabetes insipidus
ALP	alkaline phosphatase	DIC	disseminated intravascular coagulopathy
ALT	alanine transaminase		
AMA	antimitochondrial antibodies	DKA	diabetic ketoacidosis
ANA	antinuclear antibodies	DMPA	depot medroxyprogesterone acetate
APTT	activated partial thromboplastin time		
		dsDNA	double-stranded DNA antibodies
ARB	angiotensin receptor blocker		
AST	aspartate transaminase	DVT	deep vein thrombosis
BJP	Bence Jones protein	EBV	Epstein–Barr virus
BMI	body mass index	ECG	electrocardiogram
BNP	B-type NP	ED	erectile dysfunction
BV	bacterial vaginosis	eGFR	estimated glomerular filtration rate
CCP	cyclic citrullinated peptide antibodies		
		EIA	enzyme immunoassay
CDI	*Clostridioides difficile* infection	ELF	enhanced liver fibrosis
cfu	colony-forming units	ELISA	enzyme-linked immunosorbent assay
CK	creatine kinase		
CKD	chronic kidney disease	EMA	endomysial antibodies
CLIFT	*Crithidia luciliae* immunofluorescence assay	ENA	extractable nuclear antigen antibodies
CLL	chronic lymphocytic leukaemia	ESC	European Society of Cardiology
CML	chronic myeloid leukaemia	ESR	erythrocyte sedimentation rate
CMML	chronic myelomonocytic leukaemia	FAI	free androgen index
		FBC	full blood count
CMRF	cardiometabolic risk factor	FC	faecal calprotectin
CMV	cytomegalovirus	FH	familial hypercholesterolaemia
CNS	central nervous system	FHH	familial hypocalciuric hypercalcaemia
COPD	chronic obstructive pulmonary disease		
		FHx	family history
CRP	C-reactive protein	FIT	faecal immunochemical test
CRS	congenital rubella syndrome	FSH	follicle-stimulating hormone
CT	computed tomography	GBS	group B Streptococcus
CTD	connective tissue disease	GCA	giant cell arteritis
CV	cardiovascular	GDH	glutamate dehydrogenase
CVA	cerebrovascular accident	GGT	gamma-glutamyl transferase

GI	gastrointestinal	MCV	mean corpuscular volume
GnRH	gonadotrophin-releasing hormone	MDS	myelodysplastic syndrome
		MEN	multiple endocrine neoplasia
GORD	gastro-oesophageal reflux disease	MGUS	monoclonal gammopathy of undetermined significance
GUM	genitourinary medicine	MI	myocardial infarction
Hb	haemoglobin	MMR	measles, mumps and rubella
HbA1c	glycated haemoglobin	MRI	magnetic resonance imaging
HBV	hepatitis B virus	MSM	men who have sex with men
hCG	human chorionic gonadotrophin	MSU	mid-stream urine
HCV	hepatitis C virus	NAAT	nucleic acid amplification test
HDL-C	high-density lipoprotein cholesterol	NAFLD	non-alcoholic fatty liver disease
		NICE	National Institute for Health and Care Excellence
HF	heart failure		
HIV	human immunodeficiency virus	NPV	negative predictive value
HLA	human leucocyte antigen	NSAID	non-steroidal anti-inflammatory drug
HNIG	human normal immunoglobulin		
HPT	Health Protection Team	NT-pro-BNP	N-terminal pro-B-type natriuretic peptide
HPV	human papillomavirus		
hrHPV	high-risk HPV	OCP	oral contraceptive pill
HRT	hormone replacement therapy	OF	oral fluid
HUS	haemolytic uraemic syndrome	OGD	oesophagogastroduodenoscopy
IBD	inflammatory bowel disease	OTC	over the counter
IBS	irritable bowel syndrome	PAD	peripheral arterial disease
IDA	iron-deficiency anaemia	PBC	primary biliary cholangitis
Ig	immunoglobulin	PCOS	polycystic ovarian syndrome
IM	intramuscular	PCR	protein:creatinine ratio
INR	international normalised ratio	PE	pulmonary embolism
ITP	idiopathic thrombocytopenic purpura	PEP	post-exposure prophylaxis
		PID	pelvic inflammatory disease
IU	international unit	PMH	past medical history
IV	intravenous	PMR	polymyalgia rheumatica
IVF	*in vitro* fertilisation	POCT	point-of-care test
LDH	lactate dehydrogenase	POI	premature ovarian insufficiency
LDL-C	low-density lipoprotein cholesterol	PPI	proton pump inhibitor
		PPV	positive predictive value
LFT	liver function test	PSA	prostate-specific antigen
LH	luteinising hormone	PT	prothrombin time
LUTS	lower urinary tract symptoms	PTH	parathyroid hormone
MALT	mucosa-associated lymphoid tissue	PV	plasma viscosity
		RA	rheumatoid arthritis
MASLD	metabolic dysfunction-associated steatotic liver disease	RBC	red blood cell
		RF	rheumatoid factor
MCS	microscopy, culture and sensitivity	SAT	stool antigen test
		SC	subcutaneous

sFLC	serum free light chain	TPOAb	thyroid peroxidase antibodies
SHBG	sex hormone-binding globulin	TSH	thyroid-stimulating hormone
SIADH	syndrome of inappropriate antidiuretic hormone	TT	total testosterone
		tTG	tissue transglutaminase
SLE	systemic lupus erythematosus	TTP	thrombotic thrombocytopenic purpura
SSRI	selective serotonin reuptake inhibitor		
		U&E	urea and electrolytes
STEC	Shiga toxin-producing *Escherichia coli*	ULN	upper limit of normal
		USS	ultrasound scan
STI	sexually transmitted infection	UTI	urinary tract infection
TATT	tired all the time	UV	ultraviolet
TB	tuberculosis	VCA	viral capsid antigen
TCA	tricyclic antidepressants	VTE	venous thromboembolism
TFT	thyroid function test	vWF	von Willebrand factor
TG	triglyceride	VZV	varicella zoster virus
TIA	transient ischaemic attack	WCC	white cell count
TIBC	total iron-binding capacity		

A note on units and their abbreviations

In this book we have used the lower-case Greek letter mu (μ) to represent 'micro' in units such as μg (micrograms).

Be aware that some lab results will show this as a lower-case 'u' instead. This should not be confused with the upper-case U used in 'IU' (international units).

How to use this book

It's 16:10 on a busy Friday afternoon on-call: you have just managed to find the time to review and action your lab results: 37 results in the inbox… right… here we go…

Is this serious? Does the patient need hospital admission today?
It's just out of the reference range – shall I consider that normal and tick 'no action required'?
Should I just repeat the test, but what testing interval is appropriate?
Are there other tests to request that may help in the diagnosis and management?

To answer these questions, the book is split into two main sections:

Part I is divided into clinical chapters:
- Chapter 1: Clinical biochemistry
- Chapter 2: Haematology
- Chapter 3: Immunology and rheumatology
- Chapter 4: Microbiology

Each chapter covers:
- Managing individual abnormal test results
  - Background information
  - Causes
  - History and examination
  - Investigations: initial and further tests
  - Referral
  - GP management tips
- The role of specific tests
  - Indications for use
  - Interpretation tips

From a secondary care perspective, it is important to empower primary care colleagues to safely manage test results and appropriately refer if required; this helps avoid unnecessary strain on an already burdened system. Conversely, primary care teams should not be expected to request specialised tests that they are not experienced to interpret or manage.

Part II provides a guide to requesting appropriate tests in specific clinical scenarios (Chapter 5) and with common signs and symptoms presenting to primary care (Chapter 6).

When requesting tests, it can be tempting to just 'tick all the boxes', especially in those presenting with non-specific symptoms. However, this risks abnormal results coming back and raising more questions than answers! These two chapters explore common clinical scenarios and signs and symptoms in primary care, and highlight relevant tests to consider. For example, if you think a patient has coeliac disease or polymyalgia rheumatica, what tests should you request?

Caveats to using this guide

The guidance and flowcharts within the book are designed to help the busy GP make sensible and safe actioning decisions for the daily lab results they receive. Please note:

- The information refers to adults, **not** those aged <18 years, nor those who are pregnant or breastfeeding (seek specialist advice if needed)
- Consider the whole clinical scenario (history, examination and previous test trends) and do not just treat the number in front of you – always use your clinical judgement
- If unsure, always seek advice in a timely fashion – use services such as Advice & Guidance and ultimately, the on-call team are always there if you are worried
- Normal values will vary between labs across the UK, so be guided by your local normal ranges, noting these in your copy of the book
- Follow local management protocols and referral cut-offs that already exist in your locality, noting these in your copy of the book
- Not every single test available is covered – the guide is focused on primary care:
  - o we should avoid requesting emergency tests, e.g. troponins, D-dimer, amylase; patients are likely to require acute hospital assessment in presentations warranting their request
  - o the request and interpretation of specialist tests should be undertaken by secondary care, e.g. tumour markers (CA199, AFP), 24-hour urine collections
- There is a paucity of GP-centric guidance on management of lab results, so a variety of data sources, including Trust guidance, have been used; these are noted in the References for each section. References can be found by scanning the QR code at the end of each chapter or by clicking on the Resources tab on the page for this book at www.scionpublishing.com/lab_results

GP management tips

To avoid repetition, generic advice when actioning any result would include the following:

- Management will depend upon the underlying cause and how unwell the patient is
- Follow advice from the lab accompanying test results
- Assess previous result trends
- Consider repeating the test to exclude spurious results
- Consider the list of possible causes when reviewing the history and examination
- Review medication side-effects, including over the counter, NHS and privately-prescribed medications
- Offer relevant lifestyle modification advice, e.g. weight loss, smoking cessation and safer alcohol consumption
- Treat reversible causes and monitor the response, e.g. infection, inflammation, ↓ iron / B12 / folate: if not helping, consider onward referral
- Consider Advice & Guidance services if available, especially if unsure about results persisting just out of the normal range and not meeting referral criteria

Lab Results Made Easy is essential reading for anyone looking to safely manage abnormal results in primary care – it will help with decision-making, especially at 16:10 (and later) on those busy days in general practice…

Disclaimer

This guide is intended to provide general information on managing abnormal test results and test requests. The intended audience is UK-based health professionals. It is not a substitute for individual clinical judgement. Health professionals should exercise their own expertise and consult with specialists when appropriate and in a suitable time frame; individual patient circumstances and the specific context of the test result will always influence the best course of action. References are provided for each section and contents have been reviewed by chapter editors where stated. Whilst we have tried to ensure the information is accurate and up-to-date, the authors do not accept any liability for any actions taken or not taken based on this guide.

PART I:

ABNORMAL TEST RESULTS

Chapter 1

Clinical biochemistry

ABNORMAL RESULTS

Follow your local reference ranges, clinical pathways, management and referral guidance. This guidance is not a substitute for individual clinical judgement. Reference ranges will vary according to the assay used by laboratories. Those provided are examples and may vary in your locality.

1.1 Urea and electrolytes (U&E)

1.1.1 Renal function

Acute kidney injury (AKI)

Background

- AKI is a clinical and biochemical syndrome, not a primary diagnosis, describing a spectrum of injury to the kidneys where there may be several coexisting causes
- Characterised by a sudden decline in renal function over hours or days that can result in failure to maintain fluid, electrolyte and acid–base balance
- Detect AKI by using any one of the following criteria:
  - ↑ serum creatinine of ≥26 μmol/L within 48 hours
    - in the absence of a baseline creatinine value, a high serum creatinine level may indicate AKI, even if the rise in creatinine over 48 hours is <26 μmol/L (particularly if acutely unwell for a few days)
  - ≥50% ↑ in serum creatinine (≥1.5 × the baseline) which is known or presumed to have occurred within the past 7 days
  - a fall in urine output <0.5 mL/kg/hour for more than 6 hours, if measurable (e.g. catheter *in situ*)
    - if a person has acute interstitial nephritis, polyuria can occur due to defects in tubular urine concentration ability
- AKI warning alerts
  - these automated results may be generated from electronic detection systems, flagging changes in creatinine suggestive of AKI
  - these are not diagnostic and require interpretation in the clinical context: confirm or refute this warning by comparing with the baseline creatinine
  - assess AKI stage according to the criterion which gives the highest (worst) stage
  - if the last measured creatinine is >7 days ago, the algorithm uses the median value from the last year as the baseline reference
    - beware false positives with previous AKI in the last year: the algorithm may calculate spuriously high baseline creatinine based on this
  - if in the context of an acute illness, the patient is at risk of AKI and needs further evaluation
  - if in the context of a routine blood for chronic disease monitoring or check-up, then it may represent a deterioration in otherwise stable chronic kidney disease (CKD), rather than true AKI, especially if there has been a longer time between the current and baseline blood test
  - if clinical context is unknown, assume a high AKI risk until proven otherwise

AKI warning alerts

AKI warning stage	Serum creatinine	Action	
		Low risk (clinically stable)	High risk (acutely ill)
1	↑ ≥1.5 to <2 × baseline, **or** ↑ ≥26 µmol/L within 48 hrs	Review within 72 hrs	Review within 24 hrs
2	↑ ≥2 to <3 × baseline	Review within 24 hrs	Review within 6 hrs
3	↑ ≥3 × baseline, **or** ↑ ≥1.5 × baseline and >354 µmol/L	Review within 6 hrs	Emergency admission

Adapted from CKS NICE (revised 2023) *Acute kidney injury*. https://cks.nice.org.uk/topics/acute-kidney-injury/

- To obtain a baseline value:
  - use the lowest creatinine within 7 days of the current value, **or**
  - if not available, review older results and use the lowest or mean creatinine from between 7 days and 1 year before the current value
- If no baseline creatinine value is available, consider repeating the serum creatinine after 48–72 hours, depending on clinical judgement
  - monitor the person closely and do not let waiting for a second creatinine result delay treatment or referral if AKI is possible, particularly if the person is acutely unwell or the serum creatinine level is high
  - be aware that serum creatinine is a slow-changing surrogate for decreased estimated glomerular filtration rate (eGFR) and may take 24–72 hours to reach a new steady state following AKI
- Take into consideration if the person has:
  - CKD: an ↑ creatinine may be due to progression of CKD rather than AKI. Assess the pattern of serum creatinine values over a longer period, and consider arranging a repeat serum creatinine measurement to see if changes are sudden or stable, depending on clinical judgement
  - recently been treated with trimethoprim: this can cause a false positive result, as trimethoprim may increase serum creatinine, but **not** affect the eGFR
  - recently completed a pregnancy: this can cause a false positive result due to an apparent rise in creatinine compared with naturally reduced creatinine values in pregnancy
- If there is uncertainty, assume the results represent AKI and manage accordingly

Causes

- Pre-renal: reduced kidney perfusion and/or hypotension
- Intra-renal: structural kidney damage
- Post-renal: acute urinary tract obstruction

History and examination

- May be asymptomatic, especially in the early stages
- Signs and symptoms of illness:
  - nausea, vomiting, diarrhoea or suspected dehydration
  - reduced urine output or changes to urine colour
  - confusion, fatigue or drowsiness
- Risk factors for AKI:
  - aged ≥65
  - history of AKI or urological obstruction
  - history of CKD (especially stage 3B, 4 or 5), heart failure, liver disease, diabetes, urological disease
  - reliance on others for fluid intake, e.g. disability, neurological or cognitive impairment
  - sepsis, hypovolaemia, hypotension, dehydration, reduced fluid intake or oliguria
  - medications, especially if used in the prior 7 days, e.g. aminoglycosides, non-steroidal anti-inflammatory drugs (NSAIDs), proton pump inhibitors (PPIs), allopurinol, iodine-based contrast, chemotherapy, angiotensin-converting enzyme inhibitors (ACEi), angiotensin receptor blockers (ARBs), loop diuretics, spironolactone
  - immunocompromised

Investigations

- Initial:
  - U&E: renal function and potassium level
    - AKI stage 1: repeat in ≤72 hours
    - AKI stage 2: repeat in 24 hours
  - urine dipstick
    - negative: indicates pre-renal or drug cause
    - positive protein and blood may suggest glomerular disease (particularly if 2+ blood, 2+ protein), if there is no evidence of urinary tract infection (UTI) or catheter-related trauma
    - ↑ white cells are non-specific, but may suggest infection (most common) or interstitial nephritis
    - NB: urine dipstick analysis in a person with a catheter *in situ* should be interpreted with caution, as there may be false positive results (such as haematuria due to simple trauma)
- Consider:
  - autoimmune screen: ANA (systemic lupus erythematosus – SLE)

o erythrocyte sedimentation rate / C-reactive protein (ESR/CRP) (infection/ inflammation)
o creatine kinase (CK) (rhabdomyolysis)
o haemolysis screen
o myeloma screen, bone profile
o renal ultrasound scan (USS)

Referral

Emergency admission

- Stage 3 AKI
- Severe or life-threatening cause or complication whatever the AKI stage, e.g. upper UTI, urinary tract obstruction, sepsis, hypovolaemia, pulmonary oedema, severe hyperkalaemia (serum potassium ≥6.5 mmol/L)
- No identifiable cause
- Stage 4 or 5 CKD, history of renal transplant, or renal cause needing specialist management
- Stage 2 AKI and uncertainty about management, e.g. associated moderate hyperkalaemia (serum potassium of 6.0–6.4 mmol/L)
- Failure to respond to primary care management

Routine

- Consider nephrology referral if known CKD and ≥1 episode of AKI, even if renal function returns to baseline level
- Consider nephrology referral if eGFR ≤30
- Other abnormalities detected, e.g. abnormal autoimmune screen (to relevant specialty)

GP management tips

- For stage 1 AKI:
  o assess and manage underlying causes
  o offer supportive measures, e.g. advice on maintaining fluid balance during intercurrent illness
  o consider temporarily stopping specific medications, e.g. ACEi, ARBs, NSAIDs, loop diuretics and spironolactone during intercurrent illness, or adjusting the doses of medication in relation to renal function, until the person's clinical condition has improved, seeking specialist advice if needed
    ▪ review the need to continue them and check the creatinine and potassium 1–2 weeks after restarting and any subsequent dose titration
  o monitor creatinine regularly, using clinical judgement to determine the frequency: even a small ↑ in creatinine can be significant
  o reconsider the need to arrange hospital admission or liaison with a specialist if there is any deterioration in the person's clinical condition, or an inadequate response to treatment in primary care

Chronic kidney disease (CKD)

Background

- CKD is defined as abnormalities in kidney function and/or structure present for >3 months: it is validated for use where kidney function is stable
- CKD should be diagnosed if either of the following are present for a minimum of 3 months:
  - eGFR <60, **or**
  - urine albumin:creatinine ratio (ACR) >3 mg/mmol
- CKD is classified using a combination of eGFR and ACR; this determines the severity and risk of progression
  - if eGFR >90, use an ↑ in serum creatinine >20% to infer significant reduction in kidney function
- The lab is unlikely to flag changes in eGFR (like the AKI warning system); ensure you check for any deterioration from the baseline
- eGFR is calculated and reported using a prediction equation when a serum creatinine is requested; it varies according to age, sex and body size, and declines with age

Classification of eGFR

- ↑ ACR and ↓ eGFR are both associated with ↑ risk of adverse outcomes
- In combination, this multiplies the risk of adverse outcomes

eGFR category (mL/min/1.73m²)	Urine ACR category (mg/mmol)		
	A1 Normal to mildly ↑ <3	A2 Moderately ↑ 3–30	A3 Severely ↑ >30
G1 Normal or high ≥90	0–1	1	≥1
G2 Mild reduction 60–89	0–1	1	≥1
G3a Mild–moderate reduction 45–59	1	1	2
G3b Moderate–severe reduction 30–44	1–2	2	≥2
G4 Severe reduction 15–29	2	2	3
G5 Kidney failure <15	4	≥4	≥4

Key

Low risk: if no other markers of kidney disease, then no CKD (e.g. urine sediment abnormalities, electrolyte and other abnormalities due to tubular disorders, abnormalities detected by histology, structural abnormalities detected by imaging, or a history of kidney transplantation)
Moderate risk
High risk
Very high risk
Numbers in the table relate to minimum monitoring frequency per year

Adapted from CKS NICE (revised 2025) *CKD*. https://cks.nice.org.uk/topics/chronic-kidney-disease/diagnosis/initial-investigations

Causes

May be multiple, e.g.:
- Hypertension
- Diabetes
- Cardiovascular disease (CVD)
- AKI
- Nephrotoxic drugs
- Obstructive uropathy

History and examination

- Relevant past medical history (PMH)
  - ↑ risk of CVD:
    - obesity
    - hypertension
    - diabetes
    - gout
    - PMH CVD, e.g. myocardial infarction (MI), cerebrovascular accident (CVA)
  - conditions associated with renal tract issues, e.g.:
    - glomerular disease: acute glomerulonephritis (may follow upper respiratory tract infection, hepatitis B, hepatitis C or HIV infection)
    - obstructive uropathy: structural renal tract disease, neurogenic bladder, benign prostatic hypertrophy, calculi
    - multisystem diseases: SLE (lupus nephritis), vasculitis, HIV, myeloma
- Current or past history of AKI
- Potentially nephrotoxic procedures (such as radiotherapy) or drugs, e.g.:
  - aminoglycosides, ACEi, ARBs, bisphosphonates, calcineurin inhibitors (such as ciclosporin or tacrolimus), diuretics, lithium, methotrexate, PPIs, NSAIDs
- Family history (FHx): CKD stage 5, hereditary kidney disease (polycystic kidney disease)
- Signs and symptoms:
  - lethargy, itch, sleep disturbance, night cramps
  - breathlessness, oedema (renal sodium retention, ↓ albumin or heart failure)
  - bone pain
  - poor appetite, weight loss, nausea, vomiting, taste disturbance
  - altered urine output:
    - polyuria (impaired tubular concentrating ability)
    - nocturia (impaired solute diuresis or oedema)
    - oliguria (urine output <0.5 mL/kg/hour, if catheter *in situ*)
  - pallor (renal anaemia)
  - flank mass (renal cysts or malignancy)
  - palpable distended bladder (obstructive uropathy)
  - peripheral neuropathy
  - rashes: ecchymosis and purpura (haematological consequences of CKD), or signs of other systemic causes (SLE)
  - haematuria or proteinuria (frothy urine)

Investigations

- Initial
  - serum creatinine and eGFR
    - if eGFR <60, repeat within 2 weeks to exclude AKI
    - if eGFR remains <60 on repeat, with no sudden deterioration suggesting AKI, repeat eGFR within 3 months
  - early morning urine ACR
    - 3–70 mg/mmol: repeat early morning sample to confirm the results within 3 months
    - ≥70 mg/mmol: repeat not needed
  - urine dipstick (haematuria)
    - if there is 1+ or more of blood, arrange mid-stream urine (MSU) sample to exclude a UTI
    - if there is persistent invisible haematuria (two out of three urine dipstick tests show 1+ or more of blood after exclusion of a UTI), with or without proteinuria, consider the possibility of urinary tract malignancy in appropriate age groups
  - HbA1c, lipid profile
- Consider
  - renal USS: suspected urinary tract stones or obstruction, FHx polycystic kidney disease
  - HIV: unexplained chronic renal impairment is an indicator condition
  - CKD 4 and 5: serum calcium, phosphate, vitamin D, parathyroid hormone (PTH) (exclude renal metabolic and bone disorders)
  - full blood count (FBC) in those with CKD category G3–G5 and in other people if clinically indicated (to exclude renal anaemia)
    - if eGFR >60, investigate other causes of anaemia as it is unlikely to be caused by CKD
    - if eGFR is 30–60, investigate other causes of anaemia, but use clinical judgement to decide how extensive this investigation should be, because the anaemia may be caused by CKD
    - if eGFR <30, think about other causes of anaemia, but note that anaemia is often caused by CKD

Referral

Emergency admission

- Acutely unwell
- Renal outflow obstruction and associated complications, e.g. urinary retention, hyperkalaemia (potassium >6 mmol/L), severe uraemia, signs of fluid overload or dehydration

Urgent suspected cancer

- Unexplained, non-visible haematuria in those aged ≥60, with dysuria or ↑ white cell count (WCC) on a blood test (bladder cancer)
- Unexplained, visible haematuria in those aged ≥45, either without UTI or that persists or recurs after successful treatment of UTI (bladder or renal cancer)

Routine (nephrology, stable patient)

- Five-year risk of needing renal replacement therapy >5%
  - measured using the Kidney Failure Risk Calculator (www.kidneyfailurerisk.co.uk)
- Accelerated progression of CKD, defined as a sustained ↓ eGFR of:
  - ≥25% within 12 months *and* a change in CKD category **or**
  - ≥15 mL/min/1.73m^2 within 12 months
- Urine ACR:
  - ≥70 mg/mmol, unless known to be associated with diabetes
  - ≥30 mg/mmol and persistent haematuria, after exclusion of a UTI
- Uncontrolled hypertension despite 4 drugs at therapeutic doses
- Suspected genetic cause, e.g. polycystic kidney disease
- Suspected renal artery stenosis: suspect if there is ↓ eGFR of ≥30% within 3 months of starting or increasing the dose of a renin–angiotensin system antagonist
- Suspected complication of CKD, e.g.:
  - decline in nutritional status or malnutrition, and persistent hyperkalaemia
  - end-stage renal disease
  - renal anaemia
  - renal mineral and bone disorder
  - persistent metabolic acidosis
- Diagnostic uncertainty

GP management tips

- Interpret the eGFR result with caution in:
  - extremes of muscle mass
  - pregnancy
  - oedema
  - those who are malnourished or using protein supplements
  - specific ethnic groups, e.g. black, Asian or other minority ethnic groups (use has not been well validated in these groups)
  - AKI
- Allow for biological and analytical variability of serum creatinine (±5%) when interpreting changes in eGFR

1.1.2 Sodium

Hypernatraemia (sodium Na >146 mmol/L)

Normal range 133–146 mmol/L (Pathology Harmony)

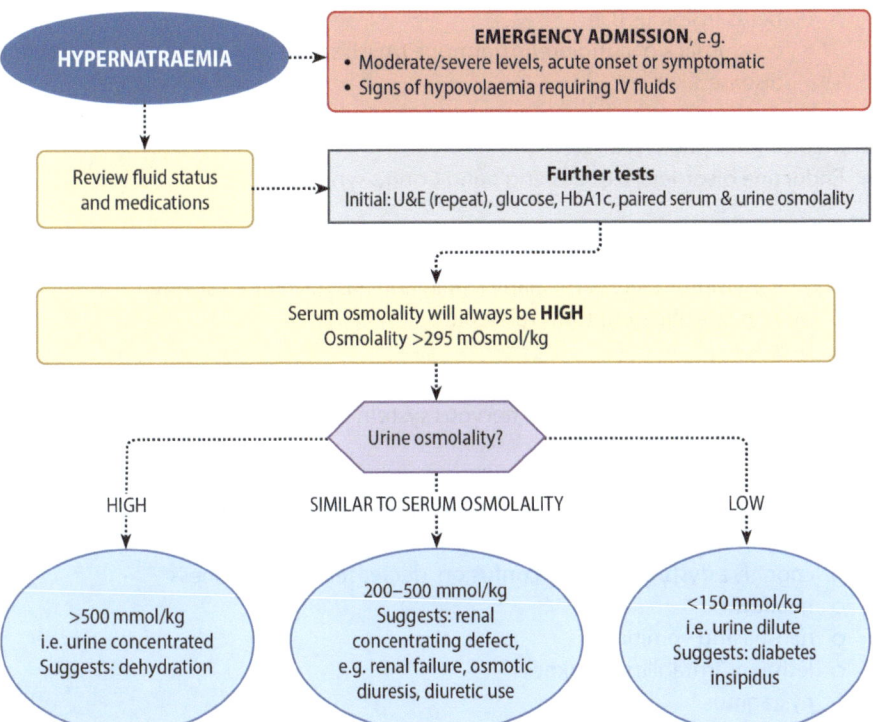

Background

- Usually due to a deficiency of water, rather than an excess of sodium
- Excessive intake of sodium is an uncommon cause (urea will be normal)

Classifications

Severity
- Severe: Na >155 mmol/L
- Moderate: Na 151–155 mmol/L
- Mild: Na 147–150 mmol/L

Rate of onset
- Acute (<48 hrs)
- Chronic (>48 hrs)

Causes

- Most common: dehydration
  - o poor oral intake (especially in elderly, dementia, residential care settings)
  - o excess loss: diarrhoea, fever with excessive sweating, diuretics
  - o diabetes: osmotic diuresis from hyperosmolar hyperglycaemic state (decompensated form of type 2 diabetes)
  - o diabetes insipidus (DI)
    - central: lack of antidiuretic hormone (ADH) secretion – head injury or pituitary disease
    - nephrogenic: renal resistance to ADH – lithium
- Medications: phenytoin, steroids
- Endocrine disorders, e.g. Cushing's and Conn's syndrome

History and examination

- May be asymptomatic, particularly if mild and has developed slowly
- Often non-specific symptoms related to:
  - o severity
  - o rate of onset
  - o intrinsic ability of the central nervous system (CNS) to adapt to changing osmolar stress
  - o range and degree of comorbidities
- Symptoms are primarily neurological and reflect brain volume shrinkage:
  - o dehydration and thirst
  - o cognitive dysfunction, e.g. confusion, decreased consciousness
  - o headache
  - o nausea and vomiting
  - o lethargy, irritability, weakness
  - o nystagmus
  - o myoclonic jerks, seizures
- Examination
  - o volume status, assess for dehydration

Investigations

Initial:
- U&E: repeat (timescale dependent on clinical judgement) to exclude a rapidly increasing level
- Glucose, HbA1c
- Paired serum and urine osmolality

Referral

Emergency admission

- Moderate to severe, acute onset or symptomatic hypernatraemia
- Signs of dehydration and requires IV fluids

Routine

- Unclear cause (endocrinology)

GP management tips

- If mild and chronic, aim to correct dehydration with increased oral water intake and monitor
- If persistent and stable mild hypernatraemia, without clinical features of hypovolaemia, this may reflect statistical population outlier and may not require investigation unless there has been a large recent increase
- Interpreting serum and urine osmolality:
  - these tests should be requested together
  - serum osmolality
    - reference range: 275–295 mOsmol/kg
    - is a measure of the number of osmotically active solute particles (such as sodium) per kilogram of serum
  - urine osmolality:
    - is a measure of the number of osmotically active solute particles (such as sodium) per kilogram of urine
    - provides an estimate of ADH activity and a measure of urine concentration: high values indicate maximally concentrated urine and low values very dilute urine
    - may vary between 50 and 1200 mOsmol/kg in a healthy individual depending upon hydration: there is no reference range, as interpretation depends on whether the urine is appropriately concentrated or dilute for the clinical state of the patient at that time
    - a urine osmolality of >700 mOsmol/kg excludes diabetes insipidus

Hyponatraemia (sodium Na <133 mmol/L)

Normal range 133–146 mmol/L (Pathology Harmony)

Background

Classifications

Severity
- Severe: Na <125 mmol/L
- Moderate: Na 125–129 mmol/L
- Mild: Na 130–132 mmol/L

Rate of onset
- Acute (<48 hours)
- Chronic (>48 hours)

Serum osmolality
- Hypertonic or hyperosmolar (high serum osmolality)
- Pseudohyponatraemia or isotonic (normal serum osmolality)
  - falsely low sodium due to hyperproteinaemia (multiple myeloma is the most common cause) or hypertriglyceridaemia

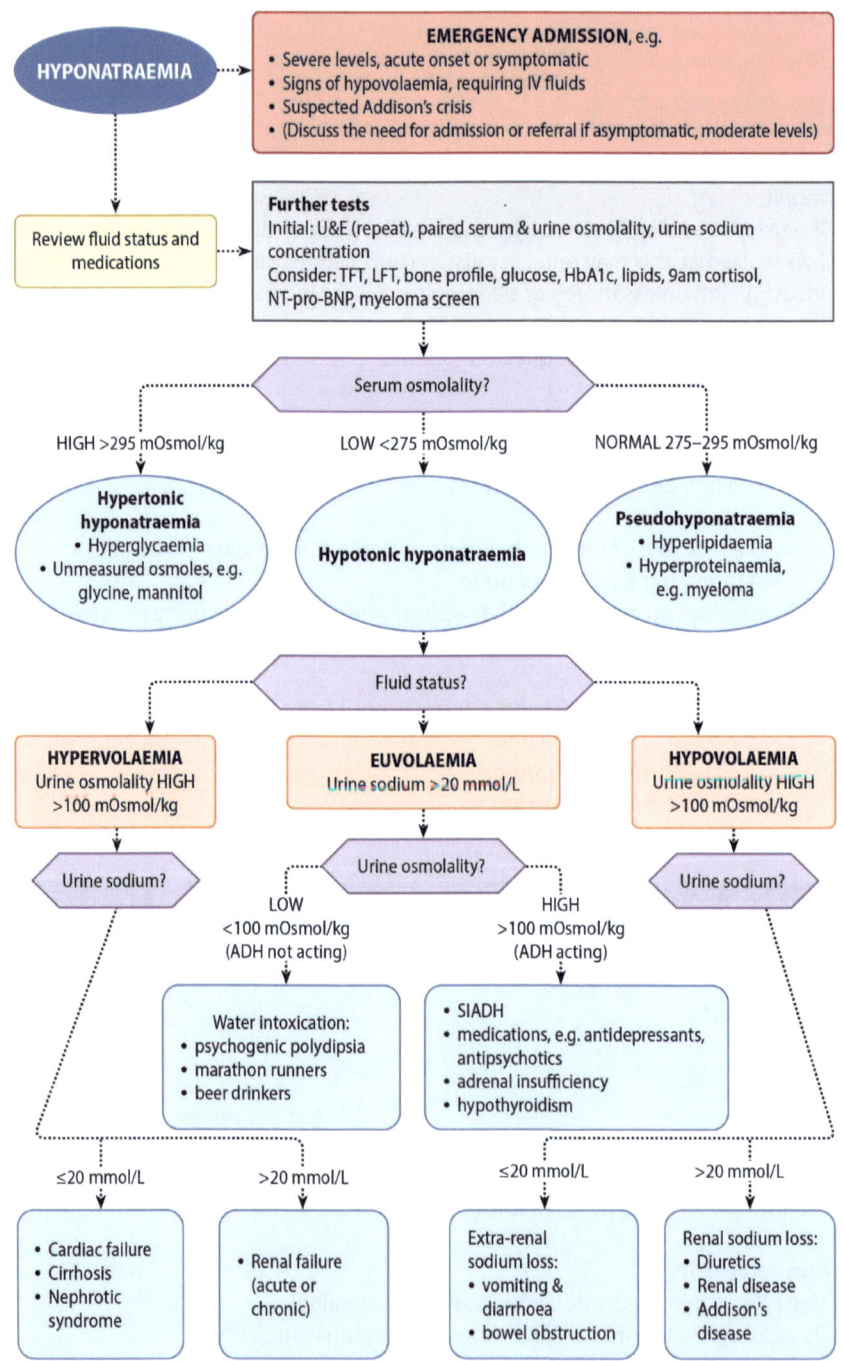

Adapted from Braun, M.M., Barstow, C.H. and Pyzocha, N.J. (2015) Diagnosis and management of sodium disorders: hyponatremia and hypernatremia. *Am Fam Physician*, 91(5):299–307; and *BMJ* (updated 2024) *Assessment of hyponatraemia.* https://bestpractice.bmj.com/topics/en-gb/57

- Hypotonic or true (low serum osmolality)
  - can be further classified by volume status:
    - hypovolaemia (volume depletion)
    - hypervolaemia (volume overload)
    - euvolaemia (normal volume)

Causes

Often multifactorial:
- Medications: thiazide diuretics, selective serotonin reuptake inhibitors (SSRIs) (especially citalopram)
  - others: antipsychotics (haloperidol), carbamazepine, opioids, ACEi, ARBs, PPIs, anticonvulsants (sodium valproate, lamotrigine), amiodarone, NSAIDs, MDMA (Ecstasy)
- Chronic disease: heart failure, kidney disease, liver disease
- Syndrome of inappropriate antidiuretic hormone (SIADH)
  - characterised by excessive release of ADH that cannot be suppressed, either from the posterior pituitary gland, or an abnormal non-pituitary source, which produces water excess without major sodium retention
  - causes:
    - malignancy, e.g. small cell lung cancer, gastrointestinal (GI) tract cancers
    - CNS disorders, e.g. subarachnoid haemorrhage, meningitis, encephalitis
    - pulmonary disease, e.g. pneumonia
    - non-specific, e.g. medications, pain, nausea, stress, general anaesthesia
    - idiopathic
  - diagnostic features:
    - euvolaemia
    - urine osmolality >100 mOsmol/kg
    - urine sodium >30 mmol/L
    - normal renal, adrenal (9am cortisol), and thyroid function
- Primary polydipsia (rare):
  - caused by a dry mouth from anticholinergic medications or associated with psychiatric disorders

History and examination

- Most are asymptomatic, particularly if mild and has developed slowly
- Often non-specific symptoms related to:
  - severity
  - rate of onset
  - ability of the CNS to adapt
  - range and degree of comorbidities
- Symptoms:
  - mild, chronic: gait instability, falls, concentration and cognitive deficits
  - severe ± rapid onset: vomiting, drowsiness, headache, seizures, coma, cardio-respiratory arrest

- Examination
  - volume status

Investigations

Initial:
- U&E: repeat (timescale dependent on clinical judgement) to exclude a rapidly decreasing level
- Paired serum and urine osmolality
- Urine sodium concentration

Consider:
- Thyroid function test (TFT) (hypothyroidism)
- Liver function test (LFT), bone profile
- Glucose, HbA1c, lipids
- 9am cortisol
- NT-pro-BNP (suspected heart failure)
- Myeloma screen (suspected myeloma suggested by raised total protein/ immunoglobulins)
- Urinalysis (assess renal disease)
- Chest X-ray (CXR), CT head, chest, abdomen and pelvis (suspected SIADH to exclude malignancy)

Referral

Emergency admission

- Severe, acute onset or symptomatic hyponatraemia
- Signs of hypovolaemia
- Suspected Addison's crisis
- Discuss the need for admission or referral if the person has asymptomatic, moderate hyponatraemia

Urgent suspected cancer

- Suspected malignancy as a cause of SIADH (relevant specialty)

Routine

- Unclear cause (endocrinology)
- Suspected SIADH or another endocrine cause (endocrinology)
- Cause is suspected heart failure, kidney disease or liver disease (relevant specialty)
- Causative medications cannot be stopped safely, e.g. antipsychotics (relevant specialty)

GP management tips

- Asymptomatic, mild hyponatraemia may be managed in primary care
- Seek underlying cause of hyponatraemia and manage if possible and appropriate
- If acute illness may be contributing, treat the underlying problem and recheck

sodium after 2 weeks or sooner based on clinical judgement
- Causative medications should be stopped if appropriate and recheck the sodium after 2 weeks
- Urine sodium concentration interpretation:
  - this is a measure of the concentration of sodium in a litre of urine
  - this should always be in conjunction with serum sodium and hydration status
  - normal daily urinary excretion of sodium is dependent on sodium intake and extra-renal sodium losses
  - in hypovolaemia, the normal renal response is maximal sodium reabsorption: the urine sodium concentration should be maximally dilute (≤20 mmol/L)
  - in hypovolaemia, a high random urine sodium (>20 mmol/L) indicates inappropriate renal loss of sodium and water. Continued inappropriate renal sodium loss may result in a low urine sodium concentration due to sodium depletion
  - high urine sodium excretion is a feature of SIADH
  - diuretics and kidney disease can cause a low or a high urinary sodium concentration

1.1.3 Potassium

Hyperkalaemia (serum potassium >5.3 mmol/L)

Normal range 3.5–5.3 mmol/L (Pathology Harmony)

Background

- Severity
  - severe: K ≥6.5 mmol/L
  - moderate: K 6.0–6.4 mmol/L
  - mild: K 5.4–5.9 mmol/L
- The commonest cause is spurious hyperkalaemia (pseudohyperkalaemia), often because of sampling conditions (worse in cold weather), storage or transport factors
- Note any comments by the laboratory with the result
- Clinical urgency depends upon the:
  - severity of the hyperkalaemia
  - rate of change in potassium and any change in serum creatinine / eGFR
    - rapid rises in potassium or significantly impaired renal function increase the likelihood of the need for hospital admission
    - significant changes would be:
      - rapid ↓ in eGFR (>10% in 1 week)
      - rapid ↑ in K (>0.5 mmol/L in 1 week)

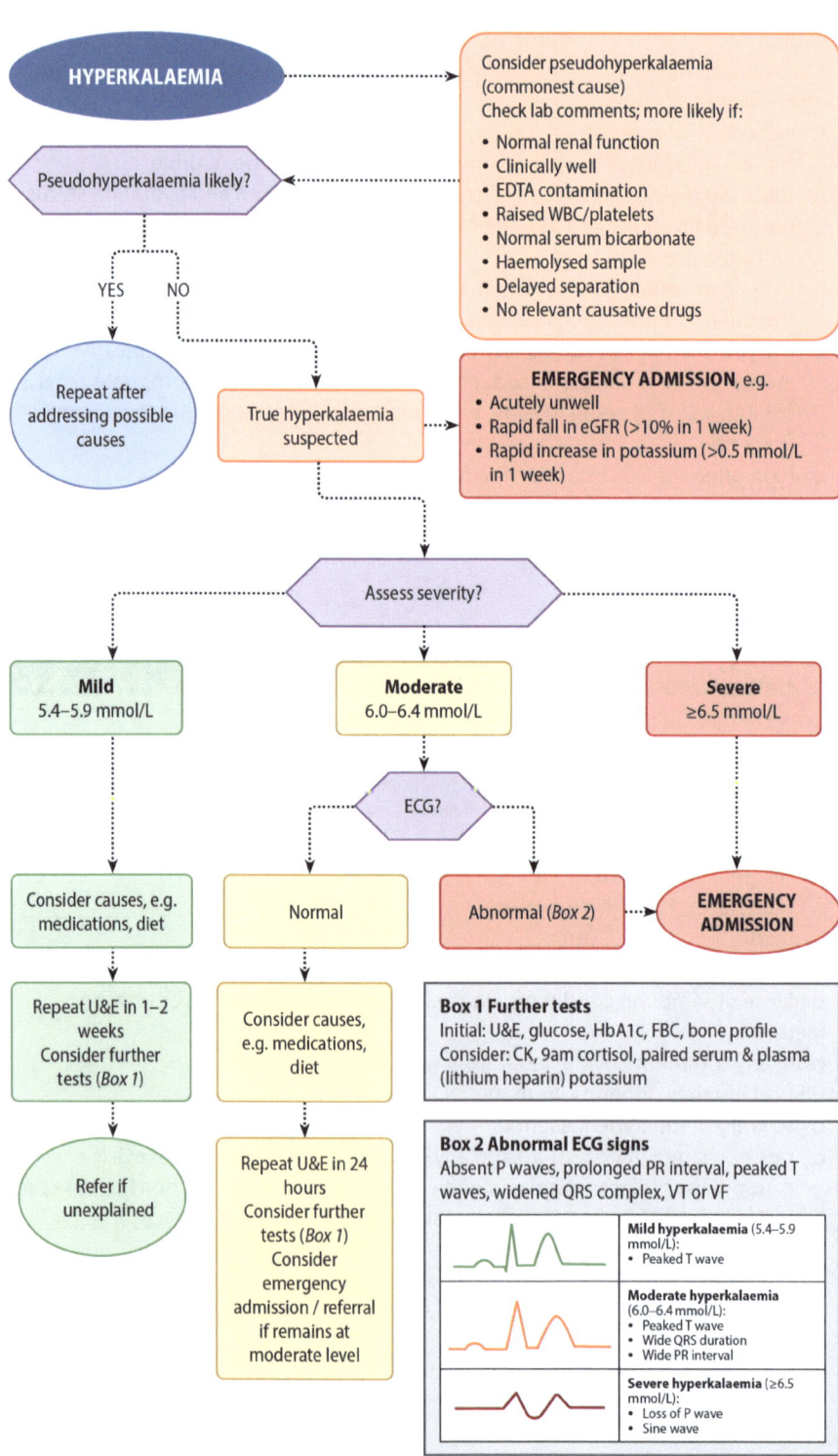

HYPERKALAEMIA

Consider pseudohyperkalaemia (commonest cause)
Check lab comments; more likely if:
- Normal renal function
- Clinically well
- EDTA contamination
- Raised WBC/platelets
- Normal serum bicarbonate
- Haemolysed sample
- Delayed separation
- No relevant causative drugs

Pseudohyperkalaemia likely?

YES   NO

Repeat after addressing possible causes

True hyperkalaemia suspected

EMERGENCY ADMISSION, e.g.
- Acutely unwell
- Rapid fall in eGFR (>10% in 1 week)
- Rapid increase in potassium (>0.5 mmol/L in 1 week)

Assess severity?

Mild
5.4–5.9 mmol/L

Moderate
6.0–6.4 mmol/L

Severe
≥6.5 mmol/L

ECG?

Consider causes, e.g. medications, diet

Normal

Abnormal (*Box 2*)

EMERGENCY ADMISSION

Repeat U&E in 1–2 weeks
Consider further tests (*Box 1*)

Consider causes, e.g. medications, diet

Refer if unexplained

Repeat U&E in 24 hours
Consider further tests (*Box 1*)
Consider emergency admission / referral if remains at moderate level

Box 1 Further tests
Initial: U&E, glucose, HbA1c, FBC, bone profile
Consider: CK, 9am cortisol, paired serum & plasma (lithium heparin) potassium

Box 2 Abnormal ECG signs
Absent P waves, prolonged PR interval, peaked T waves, widened QRS complex, VT or VF

Mild hyperkalaemia (5.4–5.9 mmol/L):
- Peaked T wave

Moderate hyperkalaemia (6.0–6.4 mmol/L):
- Peaked T wave
- Wide QRS duration
- Wide PR interval

Severe hyperkalaemia (≥6.5 mmol/L):
- Loss of P wave
- Sine wave

- Sampling tips include:
  - avoid excess cuff time and clenched fist (increases haemolysis)
  - reduce transit time (more likely if delay >6 hours)
  - avoid sample refrigeration prior to separation by the lab
  - take the U&E sample (serum separating tube 'SST' yellow top) first before the FBC (EDTA purple top) sample to avoid contamination

Tips to identify possible pseudohyperkalaemia

More likely to be true hyperkalaemia	More likely to be pseudohyperkalaemia
CKD	Normal renal function
Diabetes	Sample issues: • EDTA contamination • Haemolysed sample • Delayed separation
Significant change in renal function from baseline	Raised WBC/platelets
Metabolic acidosis	Normal serum bicarbonate
Acutely unwell, especially the elderly	Well patient
Relevant drugs	No relevant drugs

Causes

- Spurious hyperkalaemia (pseudohyperkalaemia): commonest
- Impaired excretion
  - AKI/CKD
  - medications, e.g. ACEi, ARBs, NSAIDs, spironolactone, trimethoprim, heparin, lithium, eplerenone
- Transcellular shift
  - exercise
  - acidosis, e.g. diabetic ketoacidosis (DKA)
  - hyperglycaemia
  - medications, e.g. β-blockers, digoxin
  - tissue necrosis or lysis (rhabdomyolysis, tumour lysis)
- Increased intake
  - K supplements
  - excess of foods high in K (usually only if concurrent renal impairment), e.g. figs, molasses, seaweed, chocolate, bran cereal, vegetables (spinach, tomato, mushroom, carrots), dried fruits and nuts, fruits (banana, kiwi fruit, orange, mango), 'Losalt'
  - K-containing laxatives, e.g. Movicol, KleenPrep, Fybogel
  - red blood cell transfusion

History and examination

- May be asymptomatic
- Clinical effects depend on speed of onset, severity and underlying cause
- Non-specific symptoms: sweating, nausea, vomiting, extreme lethargy, weakness, giddiness
- Muscle symptoms: paraesthesia, muscle weakness, fatigue
- Cardiac symptoms: arrhythmias, chest pain mimicking MI

Investigations

Initial:
- U&E: repeat the K level (timescale dependent on clinical judgement) to exclude a rapidly increasing level, assess AKI
- Glucose, HbA1c
- FBC (rule out haematological disorders)
- Bone profile
- Electrocardiogram (ECG) if moderate hyperkalaemia

Consider:
- CK (suspected rhabdomyolysis)
- 9am cortisol
- Paired serum and plasma (lithium heparin plasma separating tube light green top) K if persistent and unknown cause

Referral

Emergency admission

- Severe hyperkalaemia
- Mild or moderate hyperkalaemia with high-risk features:
  o acutely unwell
  o rapid fall in eGFR (>10% in 1 week)
  o rapid ↑ in K (>0.5 mmol/L in 1 week)
- Moderate hyperkalaemia with ECG changes

Routine

- Unclear cause (renal/endocrinology)

Hypokalaemia (serum potassium <3.5 mmol/L)

Normal range 3.5–5.3 mmol/L (Pathology Harmony)

Background

- Severity
  o severe: K <2.5 mmol/L
  o moderate: K 2.5–3.0 mmol/L
  o mild: K 3.1–3.4 mmol/L

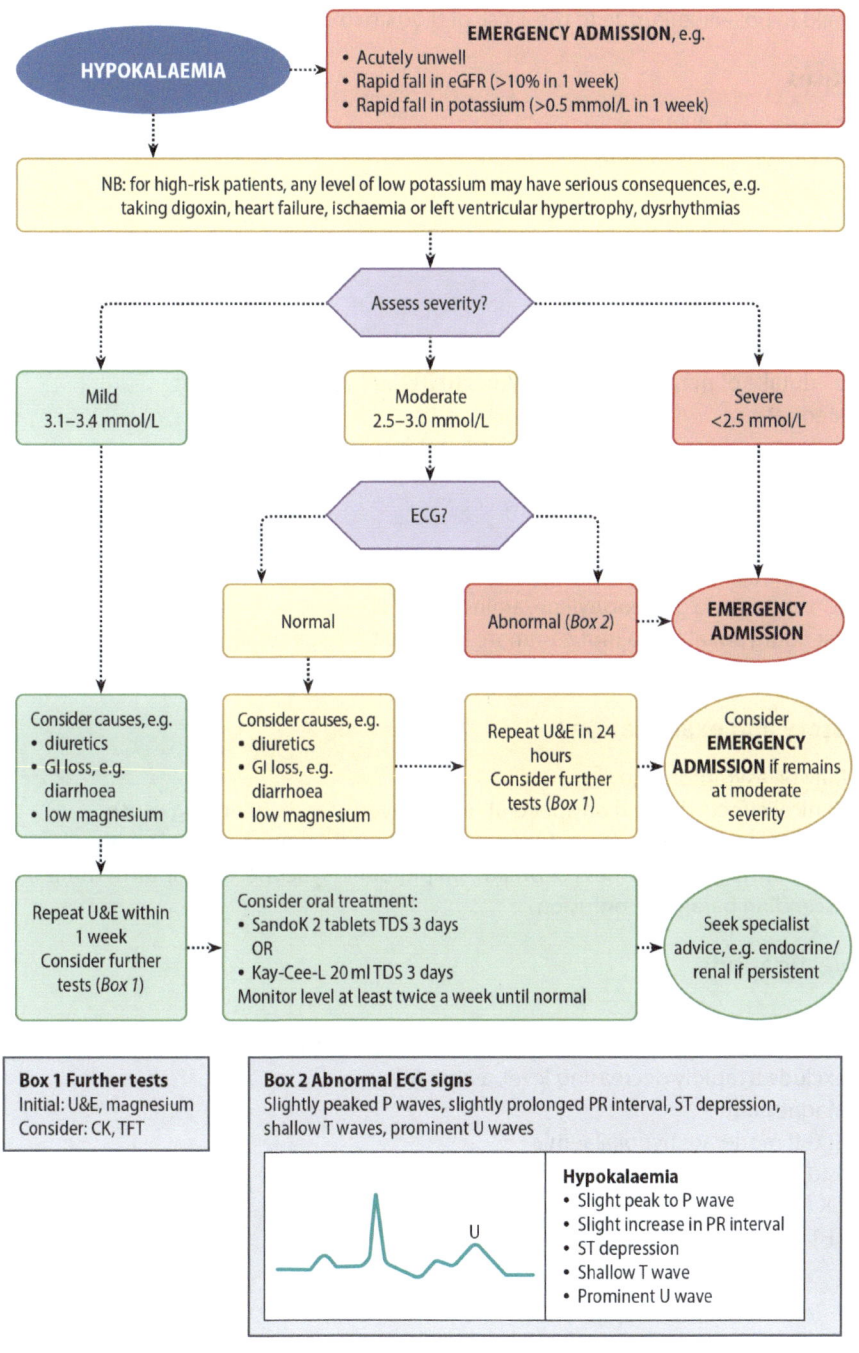

HYPOKALAEMIA

EMERGENCY ADMISSION, e.g.
- Acutely unwell
- Rapid fall in eGFR (>10% in 1 week)
- Rapid fall in potassium (>0.5 mmol/L in 1 week)

NB: for high-risk patients, any level of low potassium may have serious consequences, e.g. taking digoxin, heart failure, ischaemia or left ventricular hypertrophy, dysrhythmias

Assess severity?

Mild
3.1–3.4 mmol/L

Moderate
2.5–3.0 mmol/L

Severe
<2.5 mmol/L

ECG?

Normal

Abnormal (*Box 2*)

EMERGENCY ADMISSION

Consider causes, e.g.
- diuretics
- GI loss, e.g. diarrhoea
- low magnesium

Consider causes, e.g.
- diuretics
- GI loss, e.g. diarrhoea
- low magnesium

Repeat U&E in 24 hours
Consider further tests (*Box 1*)

Consider **EMERGENCY ADMISSION** if remains at moderate severity

Repeat U&E within 1 week
Consider further tests (*Box 1*)

Consider oral treatment:
- SandoK 2 tablets TDS 3 days
OR
- Kay-Cee-L 20 ml TDS 3 days
Monitor level at least twice a week until normal

Seek specialist advice, e.g. endocrine/renal if persistent

Box 1 Further tests
Initial: U&E, magnesium
Consider: CK, TFT

Box 2 Abnormal ECG signs
Slightly peaked P waves, slightly prolonged PR interval, ST depression, shallow T waves, prominent U waves

U

Hypokalaemia
- Slight peak to P wave
- Slight increase in PR interval
- ST depression
- Shallow T wave
- Prominent U wave

- NB: those on digoxin and with underlying cardiac conditions are at risk with even mild hypokalaemia, due to the ↑ risk of digoxin toxicity and arrhythmia

Causes

- Commonest: fluid loss
  - GI: diarrhoea, vomiting
  - renal:
    - ↓ magnesium
    - mineralocorticoid excess, e.g. Cushing's syndrome, primary hyperaldosteronism
    - osmotic diuresis
- Redistribution from extracellular to intracellular space
  - uptake of potassium into cells due to B12 or folate replacement
- Medications
  - loop or thiazide diuretics, e.g. furosemide, indapamide
  - laxatives
  - insulin
  - corticosteroids
  - beta-agonists, e.g. salbutamol
  - xanthines, e.g. theophylline, aminophylline
- Pseudohypokalaemia (not common; low results are generally true)
  - seasonal: warmer weather

History and examination

- May be asymptomatic
- Clinical effects depend on speed of onset, severity and underlying cause
- Symptoms: weakness, fatigue, constipation, muscle cramps and pain with rhabdomyolysis, shortness of breath, palpitations, syncope, cardiac arrhythmias, ascending paralysis, confusion

Investigations

Initial:
- U&E: repeat the potassium level (timescale dependent on clinical judgement) to exclude a rapidly decreasing level, assess AKI
- Magnesium
- ECG if moderate hypokalaemia

Consider:
- CK (suspected rhabdomyolysis)
- TFT (hyperthyroidism)

Referral

Emergency admission

- Severe hypokalaemia
- Mild or moderate hypokalaemia with high-risk features:
  - acutely unwell
  - rapid $\downarrow$ in eGFR (>10% in 1 week)
  - rapid $\downarrow$ in K (>0.5 mmol/L in 1 week)
- Moderate hypokalaemia with ECG changes

Routine

- Unclear cause (renal/endocrinology)

GP management tips

- Managing oral potassium replacement in the community
  - dietary sources of potassium: tomato juice, coffee, nuts, fruit, bananas, chocolate
  - smaller potassium doses must be used if there is renal insufficiency, or concurrent use of ACEi or potassium-sparing diuretics, to reduce risk of hyperkalaemia
  - potassium chloride effervescent tablet (Sando-K) contains potassium 12 mmol per tablet
  - potassium chloride syrup (Kay-Cee-L) contains potassium 1 mmol in 1 mL
  - side-effects of K supplements include nausea, vomiting, flatulence, abdominal pain, diarrhoea: taking with food can help

1.1.4 Urea

Raised urea (>7.8 mmol/L)

Normal range serum: 2.5–7.8 mmol/L (Pathology Harmony)

Background

- Urea is a breakdown product of body proteins
- Excreted by the kidneys into the urine
- In the UK, urea is not routinely part of the GP 'U&E' request
- Interpret in conjunction with sodium, potassium and creatinine levels

Causes

- Renal failure
- Dehydration
- Chronic cardiac failure
- Haematemesis
- Medications: tetracyclines, steroids

History and examination

- High protein diet?
- Bleeding history
- Dehydration risk factors
- Examination: fluid balance

Investigations

Initial:
- U&E
- FBC

Consider:
- Urine dip

Referral

Emergency admission

- Clinically unwell, e.g. AKI, decompensated congestive cardiac failure, haematemesis

Low urea (<2.5 mmol/L)

Normal range serum: 2.5–7.8 mmol/L

Background

- Urea is a breakdown product of body proteins
- Excreted by the kidneys into the urine
- In the UK, urea is not routinely part of the GP 'U&E' request

Causes

- Pregnancy
- Low-protein diet, starvation
- Chronic liver disease

1.2 Liver function tests

1.2.1 LFT pattern recognition

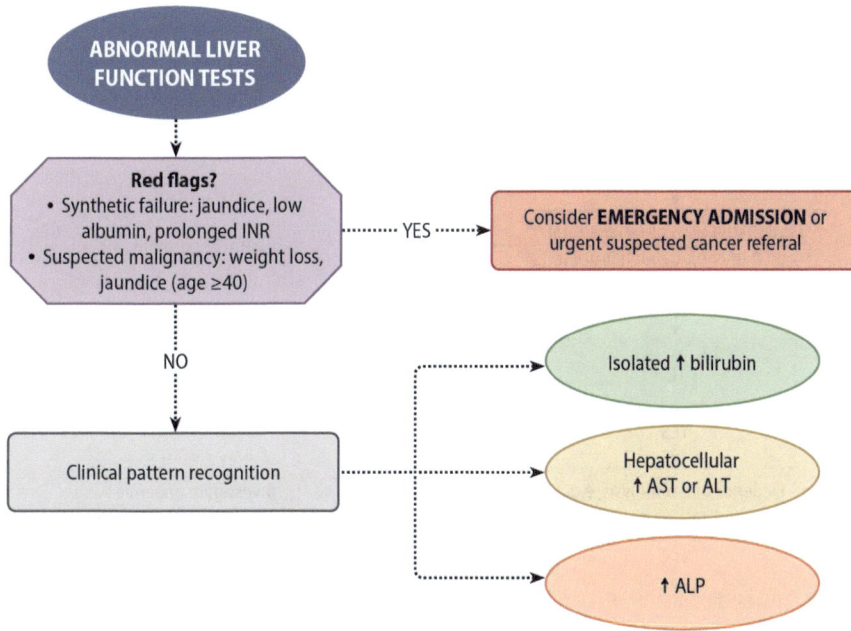

Isolated raised bilirubin

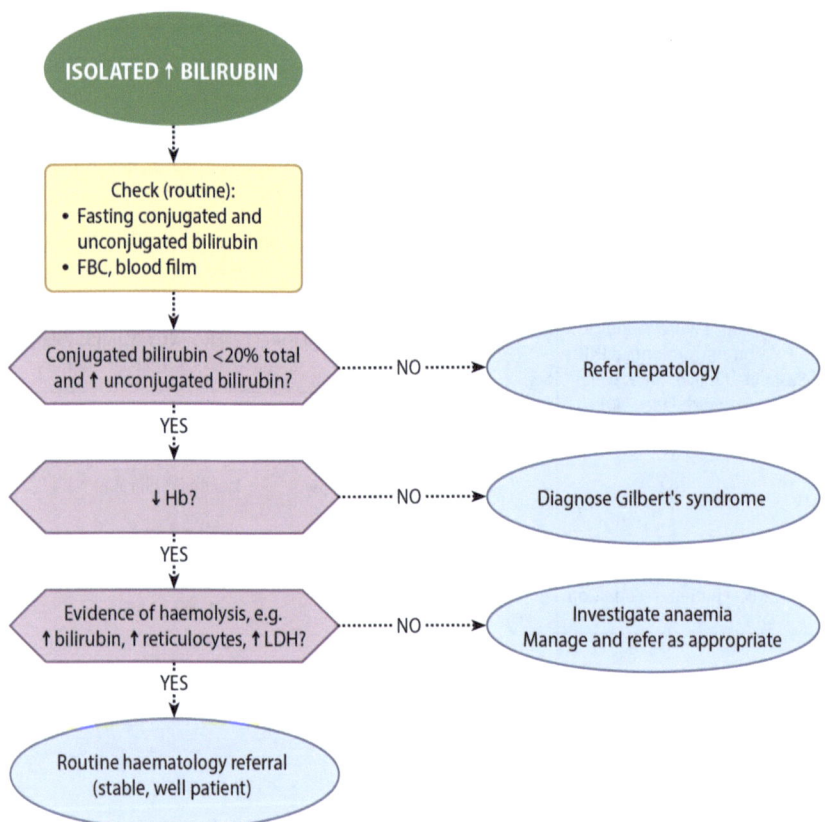

Hepatocellular

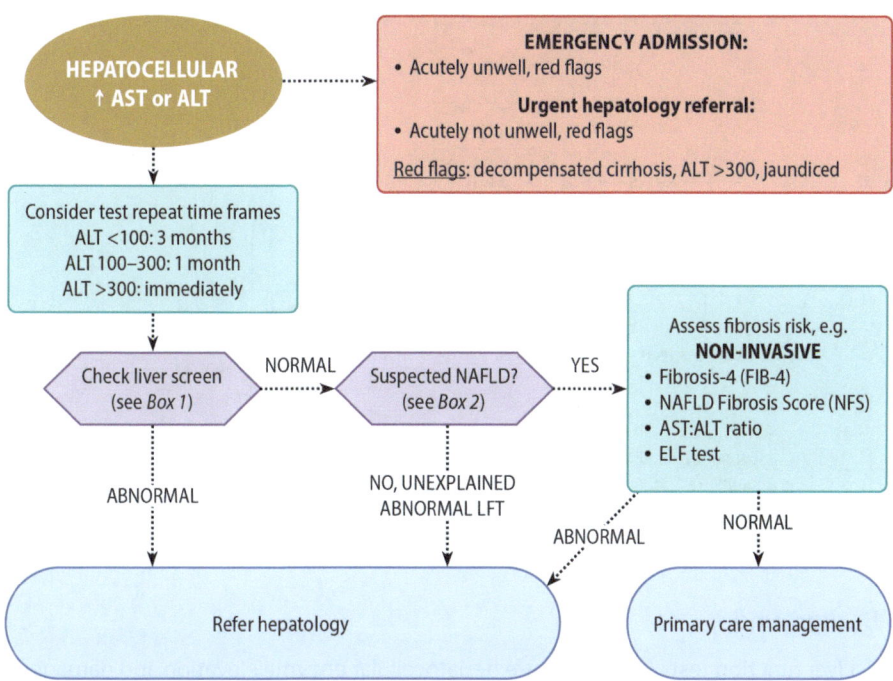

HEPATOCELLULAR
↑ AST or ALT

EMERGENCY ADMISSION:
- Acutely unwell, red flags

Urgent hepatology referral:
- Acutely not unwell, red flags

Red flags: decompensated cirrhosis, ALT >300, jaundiced

Consider test repeat time frames
ALT <100: 3 months
ALT 100–300: 1 month
ALT >300: immediately

Check liver screen
(see *Box 1*)

NORMAL

Suspected NAFLD?
(see *Box 2*)

YES

Assess fibrosis risk, e.g.
NON-INVASIVE
- Fibrosis-4 (FIB-4)
- NAFLD Fibrosis Score (NFS)
- AST:ALT ratio
- ELF test

ABNORMAL

NO, UNEXPLAINED
ABNORMAL LFT

ABNORMAL

NORMAL

Refer hepatology

Primary care management

Box 1 Liver screen

Initial: hepatitis B and C, liver autoantibodies (antimitochondrial antibody, anti-smooth muscle antibody, antinuclear antibody), immunoglobulins, ferritin and transferrin saturation (iron studies), USS liver

Consider: FBC, coeliac screen, U&E, TFT, HbA1c, lipids, HIV, acute hepatitis (Hep A, Hep E, CMV, EBV), CK, serum caeruloplasmin (for Wilson's disease if age <40), alpha-1-antitrypsin deficiency (if there is a positive FHx or associated respiratory symptoms), fibrosis risk assessment if NAFLD confirmed on USS (check local protocols)

Box 2 Suspected NAFLD?
- Risk factors suggestive of the metabolic syndrome: obesity, dyslipidaemia or hyperglycaemia
- Persistent ↑ LFT ≥3 months: typically ALT levels are raised up to 3 times ULN and exceed AST levels
- Absence of excess alcohol
- Fatty liver changes on USS
- Negative blood liver screen

Adapted from the All-Wales Abnormal Liver Blood Test Pathway, available at: https://allwales.icst.org.uk/wp-content/uploads/2020/07/All-Wales-Abnormal-Liver-Function-Test-Pathway-V6-1.pdf

Raised alkaline phosphatase (ALP)

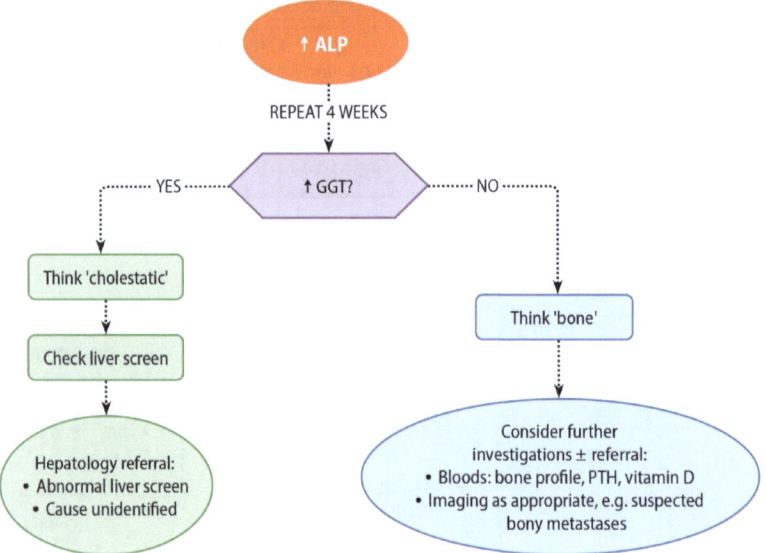

Background

- Liver function tests (LFTs) measure hepatocellular enzyme elevation and damage, not liver function
- The extent of the LFT abnormality is not necessarily a guide to clinical significance: check the trend and clinical context
- The standard panel varies between labs, but may comprise alanine transaminase (ALT), aspartate transaminase (AST), ALP, gamma-glutamyl transferase (GGT), total bilirubin, serum albumin, total protein and calculated globulin
- Bilirubin, albumin and international normalised ratio (INR) convey information on liver function
- Platelets guide on the level of fibrosis (levels ↓ in advanced liver disease)
- Patterns of abnormal LFTs are more useful than individual markers

1.2.2 Tests

Albumin

Normal range 35–50 g/L (Pathology Harmony)

- Useful marker of synthetic liver function
- Concentrations are reduced in many clinical situations, e.g. sepsis, systemic inflammatory disorders, nephrotic syndrome, malabsorption, GI protein loss and malnutrition

Bilirubin (total)

Normal range <21 µmol/L (Pathology Harmony)

- Produced from the breakdown of red blood cells
- Exists in two forms: unconjugated and conjugated
- Testing usually reports total bilirubin (unconjugated + conjugated)
- Transported to the liver in its insoluble unconjugated form, where it is converted into soluble conjugated bilirubin to be excreted in the urine
- Unconjugated hyperbilirubinaemia: due to haemolysis or Gilbert's syndrome
- Conjugated hyperbilirubinaemia: due to parenchymal liver disease or obstruction of the biliary system

Total protein

Normal range 60–80 g/L (Pathology Harmony)

- Total of the two types of proteins produced by the liver: albumin and globulins
- Often normal in liver disease, as globulin levels rise when albumin falls

Alanine aminotransferase (ALT)

Normal range <41 U/L ♂ and ♀ (Siemens)

Aspartate aminotransferase (AST)

Normal range <41 U/L ♂ and ♀ (Siemens)

- Enzymes present in hepatocytes and released into the bloodstream in response to hepatocyte injury or death (hepatitis)
- Elevations in either are the commonest abnormality seen on LFT profiles
- ALT is more liver-specific, but both ALT and AST are present in muscle and red blood cells (ALT to a lesser extent than AST)
- Although ALT is considered a more specific indicator of liver disease, the concentration of AST may be a more sensitive indicator of liver injury in conditions such as alcohol-related liver disease and in some cases of autoimmune hepatitis
- AST:ALT ratios can be suggestive of certain conditions (e.g. <1 for hepatitis, >1 for fibrosis/cirrhosis). However, there is significant overlap between the ratios in different conditions, so it cannot be relied on exclusively when making a diagnosis

Alkaline phosphatase (ALP)

Normal range 30–130 U/L (Pathology Harmony)

- Enzyme produced mainly in the liver, but also found in bone
- Levels are physiologically higher in childhood (due to bone growth), and in pregnancy (due to placental production)
- Pathologically increased levels occur mainly in:
  o bone disease (normal GGT), e.g. metastatic bone disease, Paget's, bone fractures
  o cholestatic liver disease (↑ GGT), e.g. primary biliary cholangitis, primary sclerosing cholangitis, common bile duct obstruction, intrahepatic duct obstruction (stones, strictures, neoplasia), drug-induced cholestasis and hepatic congestion secondary to right-sided heart failure

Gamma-glutamyl transferase (GGT)

Normal range males: <74 U/L; females: <39 U/L (Siemens)

- Abundant in the liver and present in the kidney, intestine, prostate and pancreas but **not** in bone; if GGT is raised, it can be useful in confirming that ↑ ALP is of liver and not bony origin
- Most commonly elevated with obesity, excess alcohol or medications

Prothrombin time (PT) and INR

- Assessments of blood clotting, which are used to measure liver function
- Usually affected in significant liver injury (loss of >70% of liver synthetic function)

Causes

LFT pattern	Bilirubin	ALT/AST	ALP/GGT	Causes
Isolated ↑ bilirubin	↑	↔	↔	Gilbert's syndrome Consider haemolysis if anaemia present
Hepatocellular	↔ or ↑	↑	↔	Viral hepatitis Non-alcoholic fatty liver disease (NAFLD) Alcohol-related liver disease Autoimmune hepatitis Drug-induced liver injury* Haemochromatosis Wilson's disease Alpha-1-antitrypsin deficiency
Cholestatic	↔ or ↑	↔	↑	Primary biliary cholangitis Primary sclerosing cholangitis Biliary obstruction (stones, strictures, neoplasia) Hepatic congestion e.g. due to right-sided heart failure Drug-induced liver injury*
Mixed cholestatic/ hepatocellular	↔ or ↑	↑	↑	Viral hepatitis Drug-induced liver injury* Autoimmune hepatitis Biliary tract obstruction
Isolated ↑ ALP	↔	↔	↑ ALP only, normal GGT	Bone disease Vitamin D deficiency

*Medications, e.g. methotrexate, macrolide antibiotics, nitrofurantoin, statins, chlorpromazine, terbinafine, carbamazepine, methyldopa, minocycline and sulfonamides

- o although statins can lead to drug-induced liver injury, this is rare, and they can be used safely in patients with pre-existing abnormal liver enzymes

Adapted from: *Liver function tests in primary care.* https://bpac.org.nz/2022/lfts.aspx

History and examination

- Usually asymptomatic
- Non-specific symptoms: fatigue, nausea or anorexia
- Evidence of chronic liver disease: jaundice, cirrhosis, portal hypertension or liver failure, including ascites, peripheral oedema, spider naevi and hepatosplenomegaly
- FHx, e.g. haemochromatosis or Wilson's disease
- Relevant comorbidities:
  - other autoimmune disease, e.g. inflammatory bowel disease (IBD), rheumatoid arthritis (RA), coeliac disease
  - lifestyle risk factors for NAFLD, obesity and type 2 diabetes
  - risk factors for viral hepatitis, e.g. inject drugs, migrants from high-prevalence areas, prison population
- Travel history
- Occupational exposure
- Tick bites
- Muscle injury
- Alcohol history; illicit drug use
- Medication review (prescribed, over the counter, herbal), e.g. methotrexate, macrolide antibiotics, nitrofurantoin, statins, chlorpromazine, terbinafine, carbamazepine, methyldopa, minocycline and sulfonamides
  - although statins can lead to drug-induced liver injury, this is rare, and they can be used safely in patients with pre-existing abnormal liver enzymes

Investigations

Isolated raised bilirubin

Initial:
- FBC, blood film
- Repeat fasting LFT
- Direct and indirect bilirubin

Consider:
- If anaemic: reticulocyte count, lactate dehydrogenase (LDH), haptoglobin

Hepatocellular

Abnormal LFT should be considered for investigation with a 'liver screen', irrespective of the degree and duration of the abnormality: avoid just repeating the LFT

Initial:
- Hepatitis B and C
- Liver autoantibodies (antimitochondrial antibody, anti-smooth muscle antibody, antinuclear antibody)
- Immunoglobulins
- Ferritin and transferrin saturation (iron studies)
- USS liver: note this is only sensitive for steatosis when >30% of hepatocytes are steatotic, so patients with milder steatosis might have a normal USS

Consider:

- FBC if not done in the last 12 months
- Coeliac screen
- U&E
- TFT
- HbA1c, lipids
- HIV
- Acute hepatitis: hep A, hep E, cytomegalovirus (CMV), Epstein–Barr virus (EBV)
- CK
- Serum caeruloplasmin (for Wilson's disease if age <40)
- Alpha-1-antitrypsin deficiency (if there is a positive FHx or associated respiratory symptoms)
- Fibrosis risk assessment if NAFLD confirmed on USS (check local protocols)

Fibrosis risk assessments (non-invasive)

Test	Interpretation
Enhanced liver fibrosis (ELF) test	**Score of ≥10.51 suggests advanced liver fibrosis**
NAFLD fibrosis score (NFS)	**Intermediate or high score (greater than –1.455) suggests advanced liver fibrosis**
	Comprises 6 easily measured variables (age, BMI, blood glucose, platelet count, albumin and AST:ALT ratio)
	• < –1.455: absence of significant fibrosis (F0–F2 fibrosis)
	• between –1.455 and 0.675: indeterminate score
	• >0.675: presence of significant fibrosis (F3–F4 fibrosis)
	Fibrosis severity scale
	• F0 = no fibrosis
	• F1 = mild fibrosis
	• F2 = moderate fibrosis
	• F3 = severe fibrosis
	• F4 = cirrhosis
Fibrosis 4 (FIB-4) score	Uses age, AST, ALT and platelet count
	Developed to assess the risk of cirrhosis in people with hepatitis C and NAFLD
	Score >2.67 suggests advanced liver fibrosis
AST:ALT ratio	The All-Wales Abnormal Liver Blood Test Pathway uses the AST:ALT ratio to assess fibrosis risk
	A ratio >1 suggests liver fibrosis

Isolated raised ALP

Initial:
- Repeat LFT, GGT

Consider:
- If ↑ GGT
  - liver screen
  - USS liver
- If normal GGT
  - bone profile, vitamin D, PTH
  - imaging as appropriate, e.g. suspected bony metastases

Referral

Emergency admission

- Acutely unwell, red flags (decompensated cirrhosis, ALT >300, jaundiced)

Urgent suspected cancer

- Suspected malignancy: weight loss, jaundice (age ≥40) (upper GI)

Urgent (gastroenterology)

- Acutely well, red flags (decompensated cirrhosis, ALT >300, jaundiced)
- Positive liver screen results based on clinical concern
- Abnormal fibrosis score

Routine (gastroenterology)

- Positive liver screen, no clinical concern
- Normal liver screen, persistent abnormal LFT of unknown cause

GP management tips

- If NAFLD fibrosis risk score is not high, reassess risk every 3 years using fibrosis scoring, **not** liver function tests
- The new term for NAFLD is MASLD
  - metabolic dysfunction-associated steatotic liver disease (MASLD) is defined as the presence of hepatic steatosis in conjunction with at least one (out of five) cardiometabolic risk factor (CMRF) and no other discernible cause
  - adult CMRFs:
    1. BMI ≥25 (23 Asia) **or** waist circumference ≥94 cm for men, ≥80 cm for women **or** ethnicity-adjusted equivalent
    2. Fasting glucose of ≥5.6 mmol/L **or** 2 hour post-load glucose ≥7.8 mmol/L **or** HbA1c ≥39 **or** type 2 diabetes (treated or untreated)
    3. BP ≥130/85 mmHg **or** antihypertensive drug treatment
    4. Triglycerides ≥1.70 mmol/L **or** lipid-lowering treatment
    5. High-density lipoprotein (HDL) cholesterol ≤1.0 mmol/l in men, ≤1.30 mmol/l in women **or** lipid-lowering treatment

1.3 Bone profile

1.3.1 Calcium

Hypercalcaemia (adjusted calcium >2.6 mmol/L)

Normal range 2.2–2.6 mmol/L (Pathology Harmony)

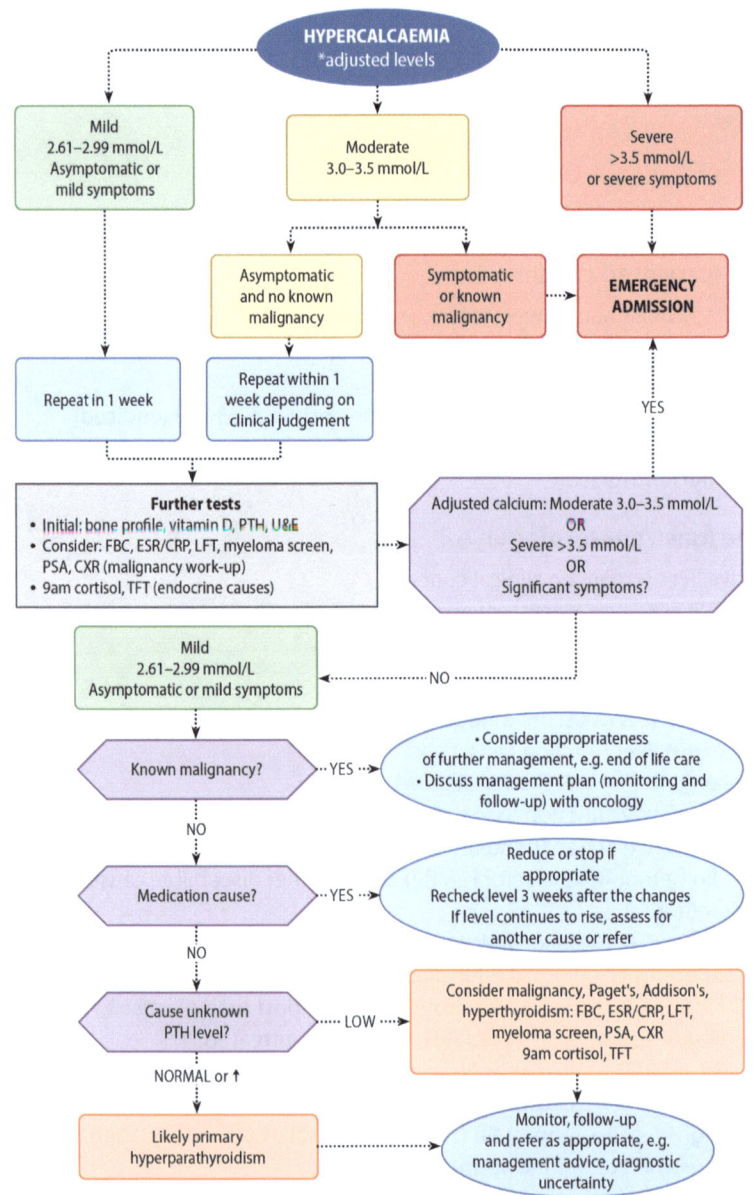

Adapted from NICE CKS (revised 2019) *Hypercalcaemia*. https://cks.nice.org.uk/topics/hypercalcaemia

Background

- Always assess the 'adjusted' or 'corrected' calcium levels:
  - total calcium measurements include both protein-bound (e.g. to albumin) and unbound (ionised) calcium
  - the bound fraction is biologically inactive, whilst the unbound ionised fraction is physiologically active
  - therefore changes in albumin concentration will affect the total calcium concentration without affecting the ionised (active) fraction of plasma calcium
  - to allow a single reference interval for total calcium, irrespective of albumin concentration, the total calcium can be adjusted using a formula. This is known as the 'adjusted' or 'corrected' calcium
  - this calculation is completed by the laboratory, but may be inaccurate at extreme albumin concentrations, or if there is paraproteinaemia or acidosis
- PTH is the main regulator of calcium homeostasis; it is secreted by the parathyroid glands in response to $\downarrow$ calcium
- PTH is $\uparrow$ in primary and tertiary hyperparathyroidism, but $\downarrow$ in malignancy-related hypercalcaemia or other non PTH-dependent causes
- Severity
  - severe: >3.5 mmol/L
  - moderate: 3.0–3.5 mmol/L
  - mild: 2.61–2.99 mmol/L

Causes

Commonest (90%):
- Primary hyperparathyroidism:
  - most common cause
  - presents as mild asymptomatic hypercalcaemia
  - caused by excessive and inappropriate secretion of PTH by the parathyroid glands: solitary parathyroid adenoma (85%) or less commonly, from multiglandular parathyroid hyperplasia, ectopic parathyroid adenomas, or parathyroid cancer (very rare)
  - may be associated with rare inherited endocrinopathies, e.g. multiple endocrine neoplasia (MEN) syndrome
  - suggested if PTH is above the midpoint of the reference range, or below the midpoint of the reference range with a concurrent adjusted serum calcium level ≥2.6 mmol/L
- Malignancy:
  - second most common cause
  - often a late finding in advanced malignancy: the underlying disease is often known when hypercalcaemia is identified
  - suspect if there is rapid-onset hypercalcaemia, severe hypercalcaemia, and/ or symptoms
  - serum PTH levels are $\downarrow$ or undetectable
  - mechanism includes:

- secretion of PTH-related protein and other factors by the tumour (a paraneoplastic syndrome) (80%)
- bone metastases (20%)
- vitamin D production or ectopic PTH production (rare)

Less common:
- Familial hypocalciuric hypercalcaemia (FHH):
  - rare, benign, autosomal dominant disorder of calcium metabolism
  - a mutation in the calcium-sensing receptor leads to general calcium insensitivity
  - characterised by mild, lifelong asymptomatic hypercalcaemia, hypophosphataemia, ↓ renal calcium excretion, and a normal or slightly ↑ PTH
  - usually present from birth, but may not be detected until adulthood
- Medications, e.g. calcium co-prescribed with antacids, vitamin D, thiazide diuretics, lithium
- Renal failure (tertiary hyperparathyroidism)
- Immobilisation in Paget's disease
- Granulomatous disease: sarcoidosis, TB
- Endocrine: Addison's, phaeochromocytoma, thyrotoxicosis

History and examination

- May be asymptomatic
- Clinical effects depend on speed of onset, severity and underlying cause
- Symptoms of ↑ calcium "bones, stones, groans and abdo moans": bone pain, fractures, fatigue, muscle weakness, polyuria, polydipsia, kidney stones, nausea, vomiting, constipation, pancreatitis, peptic ulcers, depression, confusion and coma
- Symptoms of underlying malignancy: night sweats, weight loss, cough
- Cardiac: arrhythmias, hypertension, cardiomyopathy
- Relevant comorbidities, e.g. osteoporosis, fragility fractures, renal stones, malignancy, renal impairment
- Medication review
- FHx, e.g. genetic forms of primary hyperparathyroidism, or familial hypocalciuric hypercalcaemia
- Examination: hydration status (rule out dehydration), cognitive impairment, assess for underlying cause, including head, neck, respiratory, abdomen, breast, prostate and lymph node examination
- Trend of previous results:
  - primary hyperparathyroidism: the ↑ calcium is usually asymptomatic, mild and stable, or slowly progressive over years
  - malignancy: rapid-onset, severe hypercalcaemia, and associated systemic symptoms

Investigations

Initial:
- Repeat bone profile, vitamin D, PTH, U&E

Consider:
- FBC, ESR/CRP, LFT, myeloma screen, prostate-specific antigen (PSA), CXR (malignancy work-up)
- 9am cortisol, TFT (endocrine causes)

Referral

Emergency admission
- Severe levels (>3.5 mmol/L) or severe symptoms
- Moderate levels (3.0–3.5 mmol/L) and symptomatic or known malignancy

Urgent suspected cancer
- Suspected malignancy

Routine outpatient
- Endocrinology:
  - suspected primary hyperparathyroidism
  - malignancy screen is negative and cause unknown
  - non-parathyroid endocrine disease, e.g. thyrotoxicosis, Addison's
  - diagnostic uncertainty
- Respiratory: suspected sarcoidosis
- Nephrology: known end-stage renal disease (CKD 4 or 5)
- Rheumatology: immobilised with Paget's disease

Advice & Guidance
- ↓ vitamin D: for management advice in cases of hypercalcaemia (endocrinology)

GP management tips
- Offer general lifestyle advice, ensuring:
  - adequate hydration (provided no severe kidney disease or heart failure)
  - vitamin D is normal: if ↓, seek specialist advice
  - sufficient dietary calcium intake
  - mobilisation where possible
  - review of medications and supplements

Hypocalcaemia (adjusted calcium <2.2 mmol/L)

Normal range 2.2–2.6 mmol/L (Pathology Harmony)

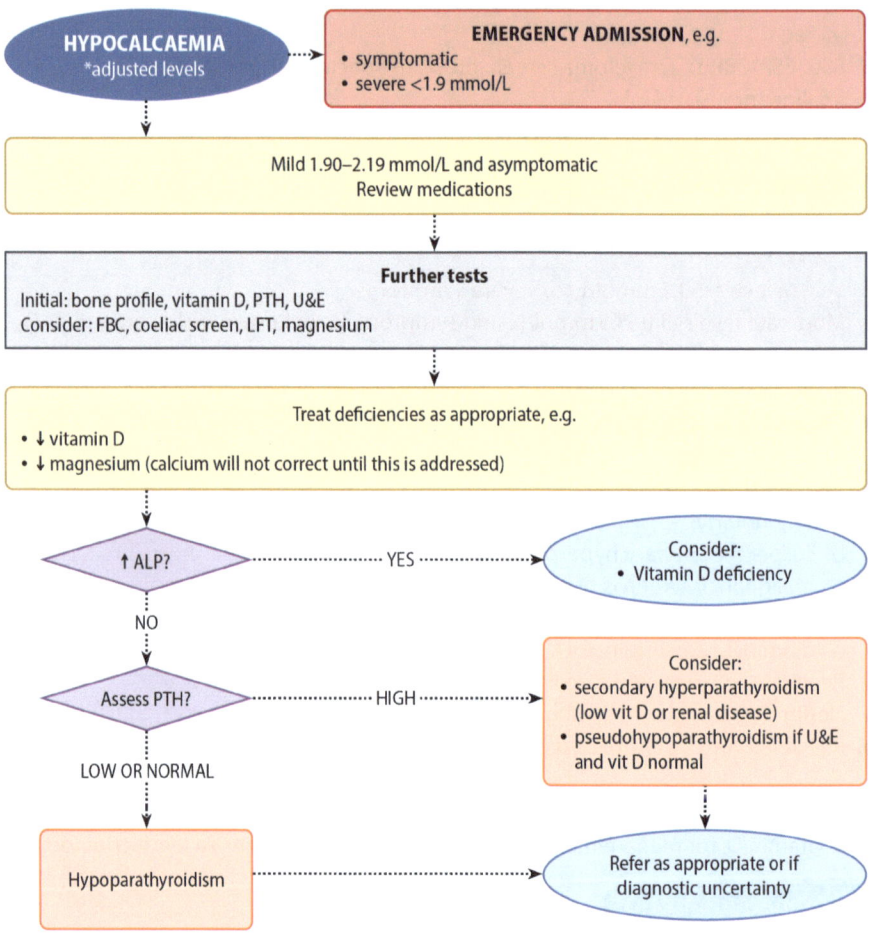

Background

- Always assess the 'adjusted' or 'corrected' calcium levels:
  - total calcium measurements include both protein-bound (e.g. to albumin) and unbound (ionised) calcium
  - the bound fraction is biologically inactive, whilst the unbound ionised fraction is physiologically active
  - therefore changes in albumin concentration will affect the total calcium concentration without affecting the ionised (active) fraction of plasma calcium
  - to allow a single reference interval for total calcium, irrespective of albumin concentration, the total calcium can be adjusted using a formula; this is known as the 'adjusted' or 'corrected' calcium
  - this calculation is completed by the laboratory, but may be inaccurate at extreme albumin concentrations, or if there is paraproteinaemia or acidosis
- This section refers to new-onset acute hypocalcaemia: seek advice for chronic hypocalcaemia, chronic renal insufficiency, post-parathyroidectomy, and complex medical problems

- Severity
  - o severe: <1.90 mmol/L
  - o mild: 1.90–2.19 mmol/L

Causes

Common:
- Vitamin D deficiency: limited ultraviolet (UV) light exposure, dietary intake, or malabsorption (coeliac disease)
- Hypoparathyroidism: autoimmune, post-surgery
- Renal disease
- Drug-induced: PPIs, phenytoin, bisphosphonates, denosumab, calcitonin, ketoconazole, chemotherapy, contrast dye

Less common:
- PTH resistance (pseudohypoparathyroidism)
- ↓ magnesium, e.g. PPI-related
- Factitious: due to K+-EDTA contamination (check laboratory comments)
- Severe illness, e.g. severe acute pancreatitis, septic shock, rhabdomyolysis

History and examination

- Usually asymptomatic
- Clinical effects depend on speed of onset, severity and underlying cause
- Acute onset:
  - o paraesthesia, tetany, muscle cramps, Chvostek's sign (VIIth nerve hyperexcitability), Trousseau's sign (tetany of the hand when BP cuff inflated), seizures
  - o cardiac disturbances (arrhythmias, bradycardia, hypotension, prolonged QT)
  - o changes in mental state (anxiety, confusion, irritability)
  - o bronchospasm / laryngospasm
- Chronic onset:
  - o eyes: papilloedema, cataracts
  - o dermatological: dermatitis, eczema, hyperpigmentation, psoriasis, brittle hair with patchy alopecia, brittle nails with characteristic transverse grooves
  - o neuropsychiatric: dementia, anxiety, depression, lethargy and extrapyramidal symptoms

Investigations

Initial:
- Repeat bone profile, vitamin D, PTH, U&E

Consider:
- FBC
- Coeliac screen
- LFT
- Magnesium: calcium will not correct until this is addressed

Causes of hypocalcaemia:

Diagnosis	Test			
	PTH	**ALP**	**Phosphate**	**Vitamin D**
Vitamin D deficiency	↑	↔ or ↑	↓	↓
Renal disease	↑	↔ or ↑	↑	↔ or ↓
Hypoparathyroidism	↓	↔	↑	↔
PTH resistance (rare)	↑	↔	↑	↔
Low magnesium (rare)	↔ or ↓	↔	↔	↔ or ↓
Sclerotic metastases (rare)	↑	↑	↓	↔

Adapted from: Cooper, M.S. and Gittoes, N.J. (2008) Diagnosis and management of hypocalcaemia. *BMJ*, **336(7656):**1298–302. Erratum in: *BMJ*, 2008, **336(7659)**.

Referral

Emergency admission
- Symptomatic
- Adjusted calcium <1.9 mmol/L

Urgent suspected cancer
- Suspected malignancy (relevant specialty)

Routine outpatient (endocrinology)
- Suspected parathyroid disease
- Unknown cause

1.3.2 Phosphate

High phosphate (hyperphosphataemia)
(serum phosphate concentration >1.5 mmol/L)

Normal range 0.8–1.5 mmol/L (Pathology Harmony)

Background

- Caused by ↑ phosphate intake, ↓ phosphate excretion, or extracellular shift
- Commonly observed in patients with CKD: typically occurs when dietary intake exceeds renal excretion

- Regulated by vitamin D and PTH
  - ○ ↓ vitamin D leads to ↓ intestinal phosphate reabsorption
  - ○ ↑ PTH causes ↑ renal excretion
- Note, levels are subject to diurnal variation, being lowest at between 08:00 and 11:00 and highest between 02:00 and 04:00; fasting blunts this circadian variation

Causes

- CKD (commonest): usually seen in stage 4 or 5
- Tubular phosphate reabsorption, e.g. hypoparathyroidism, hypervitaminosis D
- Excess phosphate load, e.g. cell lysis, exogenous administration
- Extracellular shift of phosphate (rare), e.g. lactic acidosis, DKA
- Delayed sample analysis: usually potassium is raised as well (note any lab comments)
- Spurious in cases of multiple myeloma, dyslipidaemia, hyperbilirubinaemia and haemolysis

History and examination

- Majority are asymptomatic
- Symptoms from the underlying cause are more likely, e.g. lethargy, weakness, nausea and anorexia seen in renal disease
- Symptoms of accompanying hypocalcaemia (↑ phosphate binds calcium), e.g. paraesthesia, muscle cramps, CNS disturbance (seizures, irritability, confusion), chest pain, palpitations
- Medication review, e.g. phosphate-containing laxatives/enemas, penicillin, corticosteroids, furosemide and thiazides

Investigations

Initial:
- Repeat bone profile, vitamin D, PTH, U&E

Consider:
- FBC
- Magnesium
- CK (suspected rhabdomyolysis)

Referral

Emergency admission

- Acutely unwell, especially if associated low calcium

Routine outpatient

- CKD and management advice for ↑ phosphate: dietary advice about phosphate intake reduction and phosphate binders may be started, e.g. calcium carbonate, sevelamer (nephrology)
- Diagnostic uncertainty

Low phosphate (hypophosphataemia)
(serum phosphate concentration <0.8 mmol/L)

Normal range 0.8–1.5 mmol/L (Pathology Harmony)

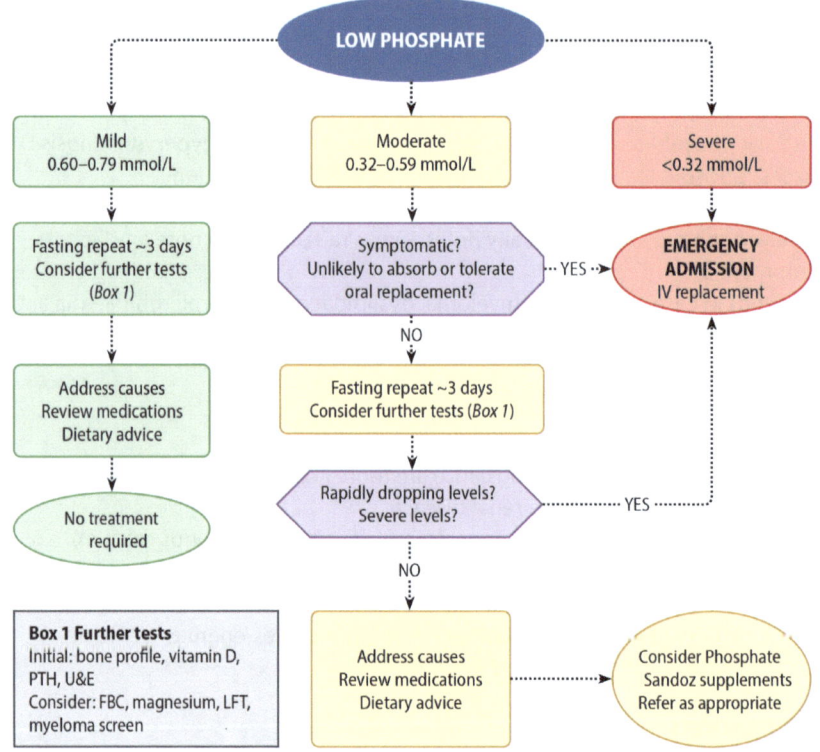

Adapted from *Information for Primary Care: management of hypophosphataemia*. yorkhospitals.nhs.uk/seecmsfile/?id=7014 and *Management of Hypophosphataemia*. www.sheffieldccgportal.co.uk/pathways/management-of-hypophosphataemia

Background

- Regulated by vitamin D and PTH
  - ↓ vitamin D leads to ↓ intestinal phosphate reabsorption
  - ↑ PTH causes ↑ renal excretion
- Note, levels are subject to diurnal variation, being lowest at between 08:00 and 11:00 and highest between 02:00 and 04:00; fasting blunts this circadian variation

Causes

- ↓ intestinal absorption:
  - poor diet, eating disorders, alcohol dependency
  - vomiting or diarrhoea

- o vitamin D deficiency
- o gut phosphate binders, e.g. aluminium-containing antacids, patients with CKD on treatment
- ↑ renal excretion:
  - o hyperparathyroidism: ↑ PTH causes ↑ renal excretion
  - o vitamin D deficiency
  - o medications: diuretics, chemotherapy agents (e.g. cisplatin), IV iron therapy, oestrogen, bisphosphonates
  - o paraproteinaemia
  - o tumour-induced osteomalacia
    - ■ rare paraneoplastic syndrome clinically characterised by bone pain, fractures and muscle weakness
    - ■ caused by tumoral overproduction of fibroblast growth factor 23 (FGF23) that acts primarily at the proximal renal tubule, producing hypophosphataemia and osteomalacia
    - ■ lesions are typically small, benign mesenchymal tumours that may be found in bone or soft tissue anywhere in the body
- Redistribution into cells:
  - o hyperventilation
  - o treatment of DKA (insulin drives phosphate into cells)
  - o malignancy: leukaemia, lymphoma
- Heritable causes (rare), e.g. X-linked hypophosphataemic rickets

History and examination

- Chronic or mild cases are commonly asymptomatic
- Non-specific symptoms are common: fatigue, lethargy
- Musculoskeletal: weakness, bone pain, myopathy
- Severe or acute: disorientation, seizures, focal neurological deficits, congestive heart failure and muscle pain
- FHx of skeletal disease is important: short stature skeletal deformities consistent with rickets (such as bowed extremities, widened wrists, cranial and chest deformities) or a FHx of hypophosphataemia or rickets should alert to a possible heritable cause

Investigations

Initial:
- Repeat bone profile, vitamin D, PTH, U&E

Consider:
- FBC
- Magnesium
- LFT
- Myeloma screen

Referral

Emergency admission

- Acutely unwell
- Severe levels
- Moderate levels with symptoms or unlikely to absorb or tolerate oral therapy

Urgent suspected cancer

- Suspected malignancy (relevant specialty)

Routine outpatient

- Diagnostic uncertainty

Advice & Guidance

- If end-stage kidney disease, renal transplant or eGFR <45, seek advice before giving supplements or adjusting phosphate binders (nephrology)

GP management tips

- Prescribing Phosphate Sandoz supplements
  - usually 1–2 tablets TDS for 3–5 days, then check fasting bone profile
  - stop when phosphate >0.8 mmol/L; consider rechecking after 1–2 months
  - diarrhoea is common: advise plenty of water; adjust dose if needed
  - if end-stage kidney disease, renal transplant or eGFR <45, discuss with nephrology first
  - note other electrolyte abnormalities may be present
    - correct hypocalcaemia **before** replacing phosphate
    - do not give phosphate supplements if there is hypercalcaemia
  - refer if not resolving or diagnostic uncertainty: some causes, e.g. renal loss, require more prolonged replacement

1.3.3 Magnesium

High magnesium (hypermagnesaemia) (magnesium >1.0 mmol/L)

Normal range 0.7–1.0 mmol/L (Pathology Harmony)

Causes

- ↓ renal excretion
  - acute or chronic renal failure
    - other contributory factors in this patient group include PPIs, malnourishment, alcoholism, hypothyroidism and adrenal insufficiency
  - hyperparathyroidism
  - lithium

- ↑ intake
  - ○ ↓ gut motility leading to increased absorption (rare)
    - ■ higher risk in patients using anticholinergics or opioids, or those with IBD
  - ○ magnesium (Mg) replacement
  - ○ medications, e.g. laxatives and antacids, bowel preparations
- Compartment shift or leak
  - ○ acutely unwell, e.g. tumour lysis syndrome, rhabdomyolysis, DKA
  - ○ aggressive haemolysis

History and examination

- Medication review
- PMH: renal failure
- May be asymptomatic
- Symptoms and signs: weakness, nausea and vomiting, dizziness, confusion, flushing, headache, constipation, blurred vision, hypotension, bradycardia, respiratory depression, depressed mental state, coma, cardiac arrest

GP management tips

- ↑ magnesium is very rare – seek specialist same-day advice if present

Low magnesium (hypomagnesaemia) (magnesium <0.7 mmol/L)

Normal range 0.7–1.0 mmol/L (Pathology Harmony)

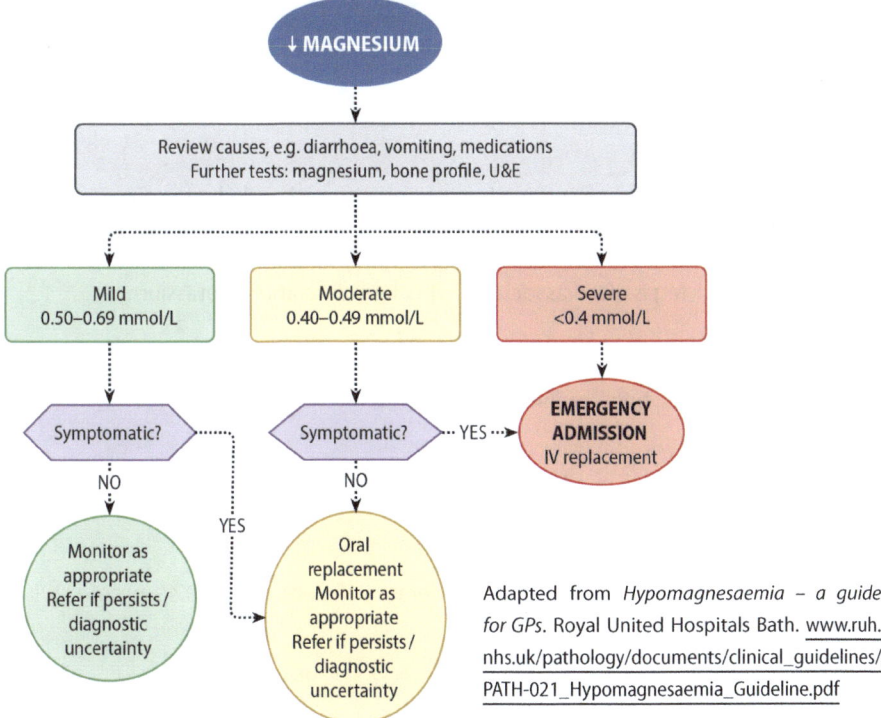

Adapted from *Hypomagnesaemia – a guide for GPs*. Royal United Hospitals Bath. www.ruh.nhs.uk/pathology/documents/clinical_guidelines/PATH-021_Hypomagnesaemia_Guideline.pdf

Background

- Magnesium (Mg) levels are maintained by a balance between intestinal absorption and renal excretion
- Chronically low potassium and calcium levels result from low magnesium levels
- Severity
  - severe: <0.40 mmol/L
  - moderate: 0.40–0.49 mmol/L
  - mild: 0.50–0.69 mmol/L

Causes

- GI-related:
  - diarrhoea and vomiting
  - malabsorption, e.g. IBD, coeliac, pancreatitis
  - medications, e.g. PPIs, laxatives
  - GI issues, e.g. fistulae, intestinal resection, short bowel syndrome
  - malnutrition / dietary deficiency (uncommon)
- Renal losses:
  - medications, e.g. thiazide / loop diuretics, amphotericin, aminoglycosides, immunosuppressants, cisplatin, cyclosporin, tacrolimus
  - diabetes (osmotic diuresis)
  - alcoholism
  - hypercalcaemic states
  - hyperaldosteronism
  - renal, e.g. post-transplant, dialysis
  - inherited disorders

History and examination

- May be asymptomatic
- Clinical effects depend on speed of onset, severity and underlying cause
- Symptoms: nausea, vomiting, lethargy, muscle weakness, drowsiness, tetany, tremor, twitching, agitation, vertigo, confusion, cardiac arrhythmias, seizures
- Symptomatic ↓ Mg is often associated with ↓ calcium and ↓ potassium

Investigations

- Initial: magnesium, bone profile, U&E

Referral

Emergency admission

- Acutely unwell
- Severe deficiency (<0.40 mmol/L) or moderate deficiency (0.40–0.49 mmol/L) with symptoms (for IV replacement)

Routine outpatient

- Diagnostic uncertainty
- Management advice for those with significant renal issues, e.g.
  - CKD 4 or 5
  - receiving dialysis
  - history of kidney transplant

GP management tips

- Mild deficiency (0.5–0.69 mmol/L) and symptoms or moderate deficiency (0.40–0.49 mmol/L) and asymptomatic: start oral replacement
- Oral replacement:
  - oral magnesium may be given in divided doses up to 24 mmol daily, e.g.
    - magnesium aspartate (Magnaspartate) 1 sachet (10 mmol) BD, **or**
    - magnesium glycerophosphate (Neomag) 1–2 × 4 mmol chewable tablets TDS
  - for patients with mild–moderate kidney disease (CKD 1–3), no dose adjustments are needed for oral magnesium replacement
  - managing intolerance:
    - treatment is often limited by diarrhoea
    - advise to take with or after food
    - start with a low dose, e.g. 1 tablet or half a sachet per dose, and gradually increase to a maximum tolerated dose in divided doses
    - if diarrhoea occurs, reduce the dose or temporarily withhold treatment until symptoms improve
    - if persistent or the patient becomes symptomatic, IV replacement may be necessary
  - monitoring:
    - this is dependent on the clinical scenario and symptoms
    - generally, repeat magnesium level initially after 5–7 days of replacement, then every 1–2 weeks
    - normalisation of levels may take several months
    - continue treatment for 1–2 days after magnesium levels normalise and recheck 2–4 weeks after stopping treatment
  - maintenance:
    - long-term maintenance treatment may be required if a reversible cause is not identified
    - seek specialist advice in diagnostic uncertainty and for long-term management advice for those with chronic conditions, e.g. short bowel syndrome
- Medication-induced:
  - consider H_2 receptor antagonists, e.g. famotidine, in place of PPIs
  - consider potassium- and magnesium-sparing diuretics, e.g. amiloride or spironolactone, in place of loop or thiazide diuretics

1.4 Raised creatine kinase (CK)

Normal range ♂ 40–320 IU/L; ♀ 25–200 IU/L (Pathology Harmony)

RAISED CK

- <1000 IU/L
- 1000–5000 IU/L
- >5000 IU/L

Review and address possible causes:
- Lifestyle, e.g. exercise, dehydration
- Medications
- PMH and FHx muscle disease?
- Hypothyroidism

Assess if symptomatic

Further tests
- Initial: repeat CK, U&E, LFT, TFT, bone profile
- Consider: FBC, ESR/CRP, vitamin D, magnesium, coeliac screen, autoimmune screen, e.g. ANA, anti-CCP/RF

Red flags?
- renal impairment
- myoglobinuria (dark urine, 2+ blood on urine dip as surrogate)

YES → **EMERGENCY ADMISSION**

NO

Repeat in:
3 days if symptomatic
7 days if asymptomatic

Repeat in:
24 hours if symptomatic
3 days if asymptomatic

Repeat CK level? → >5000 IU/L

- Normal
- <1000 IU/L
- 1000–5000 IU/L

Repeat in 1–2 weeks to ensure remains normal

<500 IU/L and asymptomatic: no further action needed

500–1000 IU/L and asymptomatic or <1000 IU/L and symptomatic: refer if persists and unknown cause

Refer if persists and unknown cause

Adapted from Kim, E.J. and Wierzbicki, A.S. (2021) Investigating raised creatine kinase. *BMJ*, 373:n1486 and North Bristol NHS Trust. *Investigation of elevated creatine kinase.* www.nbt.nhs.uk/sites/default/files/document/Investigation%20of%20elevated%20Creatine%20Kinase.pdf

Background

- Found primarily in skeletal and cardiac muscle and is a biomarker of muscle damage
- Now superseded by other cardiac markers in the diagnosis of MI, e.g. troponin
- Levels are dependent on age, sex and muscle mass:
  - the upper limit of normal (ULN) is greater for men than women
  - ageing is associated with reduced muscle mass, so minor increases in CK may indicate a greater extent of muscle damage in older adults
- Pathologies involving muscle include:
  - myalgia: muscle pain with no ↑ CK
  - myopathy: muscle pain with ↑ CK
  - rhabdomyolysis: muscle pain, weakness and/or swelling with myoglobinuria and ↑ CK
- CK can be elevated without any muscle symptoms
- No clear correlation exists between CK and the extent of actual muscle injury, but CK >5000 IU/L should prompt consideration of rhabdomyolysis
- Most ↑ CK are physiological or secondary to exercise and do not require further investigation unless likely to be secondary to newly prescribed drug therapies
- Persistent symptomatic ↑ CK warrants investigation for underlying secondary causes including endocrine, autoimmune and genetic disorders
- Measure CK if a patient on statin therapy develops new onset or worsening of muscle symptoms since starting statins, e.g. pain, tenderness or weakness; see 'GP management tips' below

Causes

May be multifactorial:
- Ethnicity: asymptomatic ↑ CK can occur in all ethnic groups; values are typically higher in patients of Afro-Caribbean ethnicity and muscular build (typically levels are 200–2500 IU/L, but 10–15% can have levels up to 5000 IU/L)
- Recent exercise (especially anaerobic resistance exercise or ultra-endurance sports) or manual labour: greatest in untrained individuals and exacerbated by dehydration
- Trauma: surgery, seizures, crush injuries, long lie if immobile
- Dietary: alcohol, thiamine deficiency
- Endocrine: severe hypothyroidism (TSH >100 mIU/L), acromegaly, Cushing's syndrome, hyperparathyroidism, hyperthyroidism (rare)
- Electrolyte imbalance: ↓ sodium, potassium or phosphate
- Medications, e.g.:
  - statins, especially at high doses
  - cytochrome CYP3A4 interactions (clarithromycin, ketoconazole)
  - systemic retinoids
  - anti-hypertensives (β-blockers, ARBs)
  - HIV antiretroviral therapies
  - rheumatological drugs, e.g. hydroxychloroquine, colchicine, allopurinol
  - adrenergic stimulants, e.g. MDMA, cocaine, amphetamines

- o neurologic or psychiatric drugs, especially if related to neuroleptic malignant syndrome (clozapine, olanzapine)
- Muscular disorders: inflammatory myopathies, hereditary myopathies, e.g. Duchenne muscular dystrophy
- Autoimmune: SLE, RA, polymyalgia rheumatica (PMR), coeliac disease, dermatomyositis, polymyositis
- Macro-CK: elevation of no pathological significance is seen in patients with a 'macro-CK' (a complex of CK with an immunoglobulin)

History and examination

- Identify and address any factors in the history which may be contributing, e.g. medications, recent exercise or trauma, build

Investigation

Initial:
- Repeat CK (timescale dependent on level and if symptomatic)
- U&E, LFT, TFT, bone profile

Consider:
- FBC
- ESR/CRP
- Vitamin D
- Magnesium
- Coeliac screen
- Autoimmune screen, e.g. ANA, anti-CCP/RF (as per local guidance)

Referral

Emergency admission

- CK >5000 IU/L
- CK 1000–5000 IU/L with renal impairment and/or myoglobinuria (dark urine, 2+ blood on urine dip as surrogate marker)
- Acutely unwell, e.g. symptomatic patients with suspected MI / rhabdomyolysis
- Presence of AKI

Routine outpatient

- Persistent unexplained ↑ CK (rheumatology):
  - o 500–1000 IU/L without symptoms – seek written advice on further investigation and monitoring
  - o <1000 IU/L with symptoms
  - o 1000–5000 IU/L with or without symptoms
- FHx muscle disease (neurology)
- Statin intolerance and further management advice required (lipid clinic)

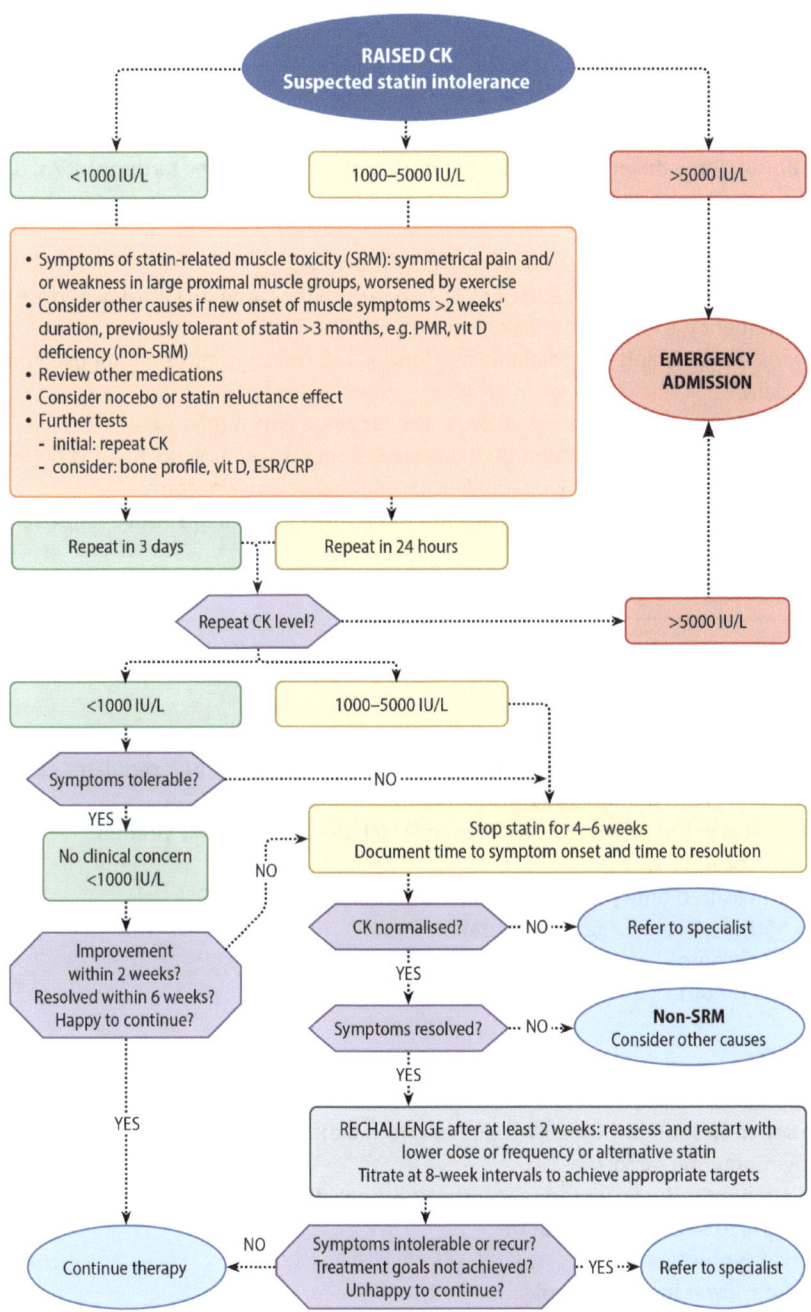

Adapted from Kim, E.J. and Wierzbicki, A.S. (2021) Investigating raised creatine kinase. *BMJ*, **373:n1486** and NHS (2022) *Statin Intolerance Pathway*. www.england.nhs.uk/aac/wp-content/uploads/sites/50/2020/04/statin-intolerance-pathway-v2.pdf

GP management tips

Managing statin intolerance

- CK may have been checked on the background of a patient taking a statin and reporting new onset or worsening of muscle symptoms since starting statins, e.g. pain, tenderness or weakness
- Statin rechallenge tips
  - using a lower dose statin is preferred to no statin
  - switch to a different statin or rechallenge with the same one at a lower dose or frequency, e.g. alternate day or twice weekly
  - rosuvastatin and atorvastatin have longer half-lives, permitting their use non-daily
  - adding ezetimibe to a lower-dose statin may be better tolerated
  - once a new regime is tolerated, the dose/frequency can be up-titrated slowly to achieve LDL-C/non-HDL-C goals with minimal or no symptoms
  - NB: cardiovascular benefits have not been proven for all the above approaches

1.5 Low vitamin D

Serum 25(OH)D >50 nmol/L = sufficient vitamin D levels (CKS NICE; Siemens)

Background

- Vitamin D is fat-soluble and vital for musculoskeletal health, as it regulates calcium and phosphate homeostasis
- Circulates in the blood as both vitamin D3 (cholecalciferol) and vitamin D2 (ergocalciferol)
- The measured entity is serum 25-hydroxyvitamin D (25[OH]D) levels
  - >50 nmol/L: sufficient vitamin D
  - 25–50 nmol/L: insufficient vitamin D
  - <25 nmol/L: deficient vitamin D

Causes

In the UK, 80–90% of vitamin D is derived from skin exposure to ultraviolet B (UVB) radiation from sunlight; 10–20% is derived from dietary sources

- Environmental factors:
  - sunlight-induced vitamin D synthesis is only effective from late March/early April to September in the UK
- ↓ skin synthesis:
  - age: lower in older people
  - skin colour: lower in those with darker skin
  - clothing cover
  - sunscreen use: normal usage does not generally prevent vitamin D synthesis

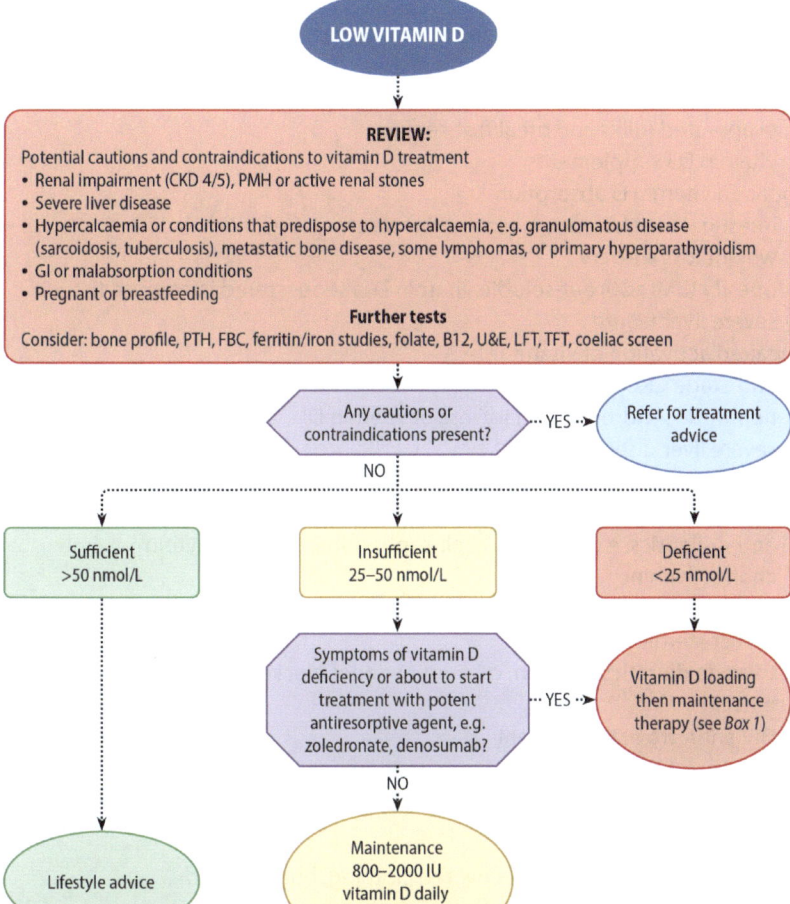

LOW VITAMIN D

REVIEW:
Potential cautions and contraindications to vitamin D treatment
- Renal impairment (CKD 4/5), PMH or active renal stones
- Severe liver disease
- Hypercalcaemia or conditions that predispose to hypercalcaemia, e.g. granulomatous disease (sarcoidosis, tuberculosis), metastatic bone disease, some lymphomas, or primary hyperparathyroidism
- GI or malabsorption conditions
- Pregnant or breastfeeding

Further tests
Consider: bone profile, PTH, FBC, ferritin/iron studies, folate, B12, U&E, LFT, TFT, coeliac screen

Any cautions or contraindications present? ··· YES ··▸ Refer for treatment advice

NO

Sufficient >50 nmol/L

Insufficient 25–50 nmol/L

Deficient <25 nmol/L

Symptoms of vitamin D deficiency or about to start treatment with potent antiresorptive agent, e.g. zoledronate, denosumab? ··· YES ··▸ Vitamin D loading then maintenance therapy (see *Box 1*)

NO

Lifestyle advice

Maintenance 800–2000 IU vitamin D daily Lifestyle advice

Box1 Vitamin D deficiency <25 nmol/L
TREATMENT
- Loading regimen of approx. 300 000 IU vitamin D, given as weekly or daily doses over 6–10 weeks (prescribe by brand according to formulary) e.g. 50 000 IU once a week for 6 weeks OR 40 000 IU once a week for 7 weeks
- Followed after 1 month by regular vitamin D maintenance therapy of 800–2000 IU daily

MONITORING
- Check calcium levels 1 month after last loading dose
  - If high calcium occurs: stop vitamin D and calcium supplements, check PTH and refer for advice
  - If low calcium occurs: advise ↑ dietary calcium ± supplements (if already on supplements, refer for advice)
- DO NOT routinely retest vitamin D levels, unless: symptoms continue, malabsorption, suspected non-concordance, prescribed antiresorptive therapy and extremely low vitamin D at baseline, needing sequential doses of a potent antiresorptive agent (zoledronate, denosumab or teriparatide)
  - Check after at least 3–6 months

Adapted from CKS NICE (revised 2022) *Vitamin D deficiency in adults.* https://cks.nice.org.uk/topics/vitamin-d-deficiency-in-adults/

- Dietary sources:
  - o egg yolk, oily fish (such as salmon, mackerel, herring and sardines), wild mushrooms, red meat, liver and kidney
  - o vitamin D-fortified foods: most margarines and fat spreads, some dried or evaporated milks and breakfast cereals
  - o vitamin D3 supplements
- Impaired vitamin D absorption:
  - o intestinal malabsorption, e.g. coeliac disease, cystic fibrosis, IBD
  - o weight loss surgery
  - o obesity (BMI >30) (fat-soluble vitamin D is sequestered in adipose tissue)
  - o severe liver failure
- Impaired activation of vitamin D:
  - o end-stage CKD
  - o nephrotic syndrome (urinary loss of vitamin D)
  - o severe liver disease
- Medications:
  - o reduced fat absorption, e.g. orlistat
  - o anti-epileptics, e.g. carbamazepine, phenobarbital, phenytoin
  - o cholestyramine
  - o rifampicin
  - o corticosteroids
  - o thiazide diuretics, digoxin, calcium-channel blockers
  - o antacids
  - o HIV antiretroviral treatment

History and examination

- Age ≥65 (higher risk)
- Sun exposure levels, e.g. fully-covered clothing, housebound
- Ethnicity: darker skin pigmentation
- Malabsorption: bowel disorder, weight loss surgery
- Chronic disease: liver failure, CKD
- Medications
- Obesity
- Pregnancy and breastfeeding
- Musculoskeletal symptoms, e.g. chronic widespread pain, proximal muscle weakness
- Bone disease, e.g. osteomalacia, osteoporosis
  - o correction of vitamin D deficiency is needed prior to specific treatments, e.g. zoledronate, denosumab

Investigations

- Consider:
  - bone profile, PTH (assess for a disorder of bone mineralisation, e.g. osteomalacia)
  - FBC, ferritin/iron studies, folate, vitamin B12
  - U&E, LFT, TFT
  - coeliac screen

Referral

Routine (relevant specialty)

- Refer for advice before starting high-dose vitamin D if:
  - hypercalcaemic or has conditions that predispose to it ($\uparrow$ risk vitamin D toxicity):
    - granulomatous disease (sarcoidosis, tuberculosis)
    - metastatic bone disease
    - some lymphomas
    - primary hyperparathyroidism
  - GI or malabsorption disorder resulting in an inability to maintain adequate vitamin D status (intensive high-dose replacement or maintenance treatment may be needed under specialist supervision)
  - PMH or active renal stones (risk of vitamin D toxicity causing hypercalciuria and renal stone disease)
  - severe liver disease or end-stage CKD (specialist treatment with activated vitamin D metabolites may be needed)
  - pregnant or breastfeeding

GP management tips

- Preparation of choice: oral vitamin D3
- Follow local formulary advice and prescribe specific brands
- If the person is vegan, has a peanut or soya allergy, or has halal or kosher diet requirements, check preparation contents
- Assess the need for calcium supplements
  - assess dietary calcium and consider using an online calcium calculator, e.g. from Centre for Genomic & Experimental Medicine (CGEM) (https://webapps.igc.ed.ac.uk/world/research/rheumatological/calcium-calculator)
  - if there is inadequate calcium intake <700 mg daily (or <1000 mg daily if the person has osteoporosis), advise to $\uparrow$ dietary calcium intake
  - consider calcium supplements if unable or unwilling to $\uparrow$ dietary calcium
    - NB: combination calcium and vitamin D preparations (e.g. Calcichew D3) are *not* recommended for people needing high-dose vitamin D treatment, as they contain very low levels of vitamin D (200–400 IU per tablet) and may increase the risk of hypercalcaemia

1.6 Stool

1.6.1 Faecal immunochemical test (FIT)

Normal range <10 μg Hb/g faeces (NICE)

Background

- A newer form of faecal occult blood testing
- Detects small amounts of blood in stool samples using antibodies specific to human haemoglobin

Indication for test

- Recommended to guide referral for suspected colorectal cancer in adults:
  o with an abdominal mass, *or*
  o with a change in bowel habit, *or*
  o with iron-deficiency anaemia, *or*
  o aged ≥40 with unexplained weight loss and abdominal pain, *or*
  o aged <50 with rectal bleeding and either unexplained:
    ▪ abdominal pain
    ▪ weight loss, *or*
  o aged ≥50 with any unexplained:
    ▪ rectal bleeding
    ▪ abdominal pain
    ▪ weight loss, *or*
  o aged ≥60 with anaemia even in the absence of iron deficiency
- FIT should be offered even if the person has previously had a negative FIT result through the NHS bowel screening programme
  o NB: the thresholds for a positive result are much higher for the tests done by NHS bowel screening programmes (ranging from 80 to 150 μg Hb/g faeces); thus a recent negative screening test cannot be used to exclude colorectal cancer in someone who later attends with lower GI symptoms
- **Do not** offer the test to people with a rectal mass, an unexplained anal mass or unexplained anal ulceration before referral is considered

Interpretation

- Refer adults using a suspected cancer pathway referral for colorectal cancer if they have a FIT result of ≥10 μg Hb/g faeces
- For people who have not returned a faecal sample or who have a FIT result <10 μg Hb/g faeces:
  o safety-netting processes should be in place
  o referral to an appropriate secondary care pathway should not be delayed if there is strong clinical concern of cancer because of ongoing unexplained symptoms, e.g. abdominal mass

1.6.2 Faecal calprotectin (FC)

Normal range: no absolute cut-off for normal – see below
*Check local pathways for referral cut-offs and criteria

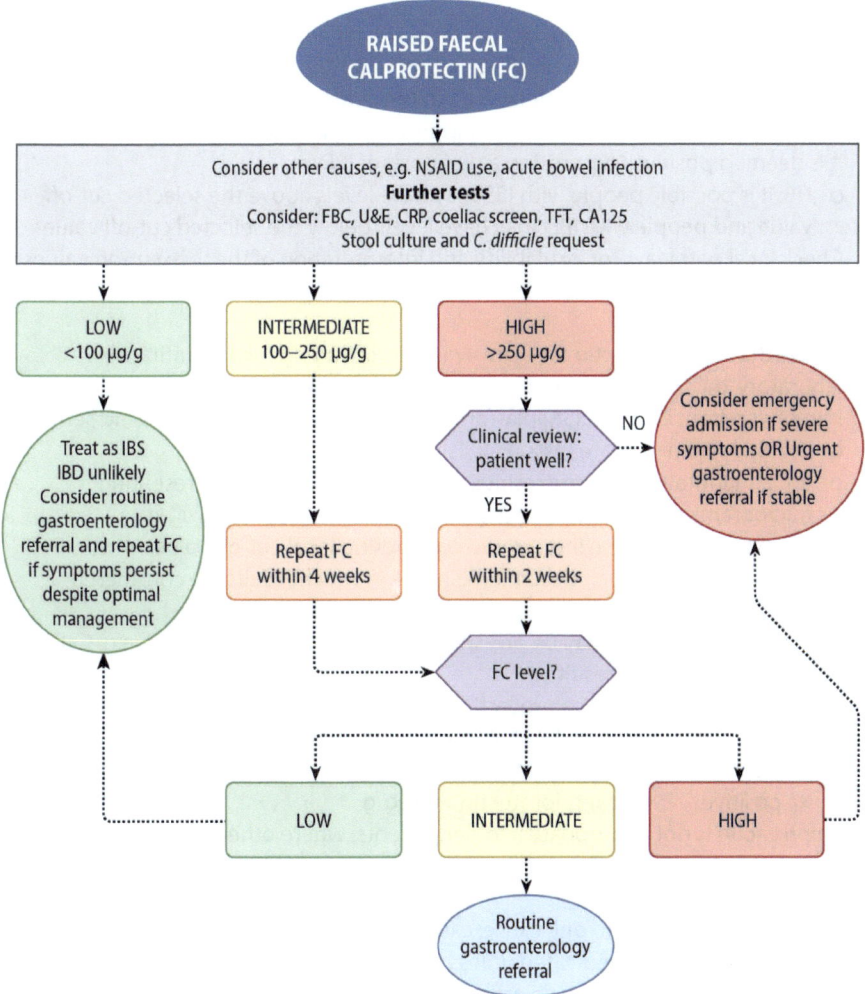

An example guide to managing raised faecal calprotectin – ensure you follow local guidance / cut-off values, as they may vary to those stated here.

Adapted from: Royal United Hospitals Bath NHS Foundation Trust (2023) *Faecal calprotectin pathway for primary care.* www.ruh.nhs.uk/pathology/documents/clinical_guidelines/PATH-013_Faecal_Calprotectin_Pathway_for_Primary_Care.pdf and *Faecal calprotectin in primary care as a decision diagnostic for inflammatory bowel disease and irritable bowel syndrome.* www.nice.org.uk/guidance/dg11/resources/endorsed-resource-consensus-paper-pdf-4595859614

Background

- Clinical differentiation between bowel inflammatory disorders (such as IBD) and functional disorders (such as irritable bowel syndrome (IBS)) can be difficult
- Blood tests, e.g. FBC, CRP lack sensitivity and specificity, but colonoscopy is invasive, expensive and not risk-free
- Faecal calprotectin is a useful biomarker of gut inflammation where the level is proportional to the degree of inflammation
- This test result needs to be interpreted in the context of a 'cut-off value', below which the test is deemed negative (supporting a diagnosis of IBS) and above which it is deemed positive (supporting a diagnosis of IBD)
  - o NB: it is possible people with IBS may have levels above the selected cut-off value and people with IBD may have levels below the selected cut-off value
- Check local pathways for availability and interpretation of the test; cut-off values for specific management options and when to refer may vary according to locality and which assay is used
- Several faecal calprotectin tests are available, including fully quantitative laboratory-based technologies (many of which use an enzyme-linked immunosorbent assay (ELISA) platform), fully quantitative rapid tests and semi-quantitative point-of-care tests (POCTs)
  - o for a quantitative test, the result is often a single number representing micrograms of calprotectin per gram of stool sample, e.g. 15 µg/g
  - o this would need to be interpreted considering local cut-off values
  - o cut-off values can include a middle range in which results are considered indeterminate
  - o some cut-off values may be pre-specified in the design of the test, e.g. CalDetect reports one of four results:
    - negative: faecal calprotectin undetectable
    - negative: faecal calprotectin ≤15 µg/g
    - positive: faecal calprotectin 16–60 µg/g
    - positive: faecal calprotectin >60 µg/g
- Calprotectin is not appropriate in older patients, where other diagnoses such as colonic polyps / malignancy are more common: check the local age-cut off for use, e.g. >45–50 years
- The test is not specific to one cause: causes of ↑ levels include acute infective diarrhoea (testing not indicated unless new GI symptoms persist for at least 4 weeks); bloody diarrhoea; diverticulitis; cancer; NSAID and PPI use (stop 4 weeks prior to testing); coeliac disease; cirrhosis; IBD

Indication for test

- Help distinguish between IBS and IBD:
  - o in primary and secondary care,
  - o in adults (check local upper limit of age to test),

- o with recent-onset lower GI symptoms,
- o where cancer is not suspected,
- o for whom specialist assessment is being considered, and
- o appropriate quality assurance processes and locally agreed care pathways are in place for the testing

Interpretation

- Check local protocols for cut-offs and interpretation; example ranges used in the flowchart are:
  - o low   <100 µg/g
  - o intermediate   100–250 µg/g
  - o high   >250 µg/g
- If strong clinical suspicion of IBD remains following negative faecal calprotectin, then referral to gastroenterology should be considered
- Initial 'low'
  - o treat as IBS; IBD unlikely
  - o consider routine gastroenterology referral and repeat FC if symptoms persist despite optimal management
- Initial 'intermediate'
  - o repeat within 4 weeks
    - if 'low'
      - – treat as IBS; IBD unlikely
      - – consider routine gastroenterology referral and repeat FC if symptoms persist despite optimal management
    - if 'intermediate': routine gastroenterology referral
    - if 'high': urgent gastroenterology referral
- Initial 'high'
  - o clinically assess patient
    - if unwell, consider admission if severe symptoms or urgent gastroenterology referral if stable
    - if well, repeat FC within 2 weeks
      - – if 'low'
        - treat as IBS; IBD unlikely
        - consider routine gastroenterology referral and repeat FC if symptoms persist despite optimal management
      - – if 'intermediate': routine gastroenterology referral
      - – if 'high': urgent gastroenterology referral

GP management tips

- Consider result with other relevant tests:
  - o FBC, U&E, CRP, coeliac screen, TFT, CA125
  - o stool culture and C. difficile request

1.6.3 Faecal elastase

Normal exocrine pancreatic function: >200 µg/g (Siemens)

Background

- More likely to be requested by secondary care in suspected exocrine pancreatic insufficiency, symptoms of which include steatorrhoea, weight loss, abdominal discomfort and malnutrition
- Causes include chronic pancreatitis, pancreatic cancer or surgery

Indication for test

- Investigation of suspected exocrine pancreatic insufficiency

Interpretation

- Spurious result may occur with watery diarrhoea
- Normal exocrine pancreatic sufficiency: >200 µg/g
- Moderate–mild exocrine pancreatic insufficiency: 100–200 µg/g (refer)
- Severe exocrine pancreatic insufficiency: <100 µg/g (refer)

GP management tips

- If abnormal, refer to gastroenterology and dietitian for further assessment/investigation and management, e.g. pancreatic enzyme replacement therapy

1.7 Urine

1.7.1 Urine albumin:creatinine ratio (ACR) and urine protein:creatinine ratio (PCR)

Urine ACR Normal range <3 mg/mmol (Siemens)
Urine PCR Normal range <50 mg/mmol

Background

- Proteinuria is an important indicator of kidney disease and its risk of progression
- ACR is the preferred test because of the greater sensitivity for low proteinuria levels
- When ACR is ≥70 mg/mmol, PCR can be used as an alternative
- Do not use a urine dipstick to test for proteinuria: if unexplained proteinuria is an incidental finding on a reagent strip, test eGFR, creatinine and ACR
- ACR 30 mg/mmol = PCR 50 mg/mmol = urinary protein excretion 0.5 g/24 hours
- ACR 70 mg/mmol = PCR 100 mg/mmol = urinary protein excretion 1 g/24 hours

Indications for test

- Diabetes
- Hypertension
- Gout
- Previous AKI
- Vascular disease, e.g. cardiovascular, peripheral or cerebrovascular
- Structural renal tract disease, recurrent kidney stones, prostatic hypertrophy
- Multisystem diseases with potential kidney involvement, e.g. SLE
- FHx of end-stage kidney disease or hereditary kidney disease
- Incidental findings of haematuria or proteinuria on urine dip test
- Use of nephrotoxic drugs, e.g. long-term NSAID use, penicillamine

Interpretation

- Results can be affected by:
  - physiological factors, e.g. erect posture, exercise, acute diuresis
  - false positive results may occur, e.g. menstrual or seminal fluid, UTI
- Early morning samples are preferred
- ACR should be interpreted alongside eGFR to determine CKD staging and guide frequency of follow-up
- Regard a confirmed ACR of ≥3 mg/mmol as clinically important proteinuria
- High urine protein but normal ACR:
  - urine ACR is specific for albumin. Urine contains other proteins, e.g. low molecular weight immunoglobulins (including IgA and light chains) which may account for high urine protein but a normal ACR in conditions such as myeloma
- Classification

ACR category	Level
A1 normal to mildly increased	<3 mg/mmol
A2 moderately increased	3–30 mg/mmol
A3 severely increased	>30 mg/mmol

Adapted from CKS NICE (revised 2025) *CKD*. https://cks.nice.org.uk/topics/chronic-kidney-disease/diagnosis/initial-investigations

- Management
  - initial urine ACR management
  - ongoing urine ACR management: see flowchart on following page

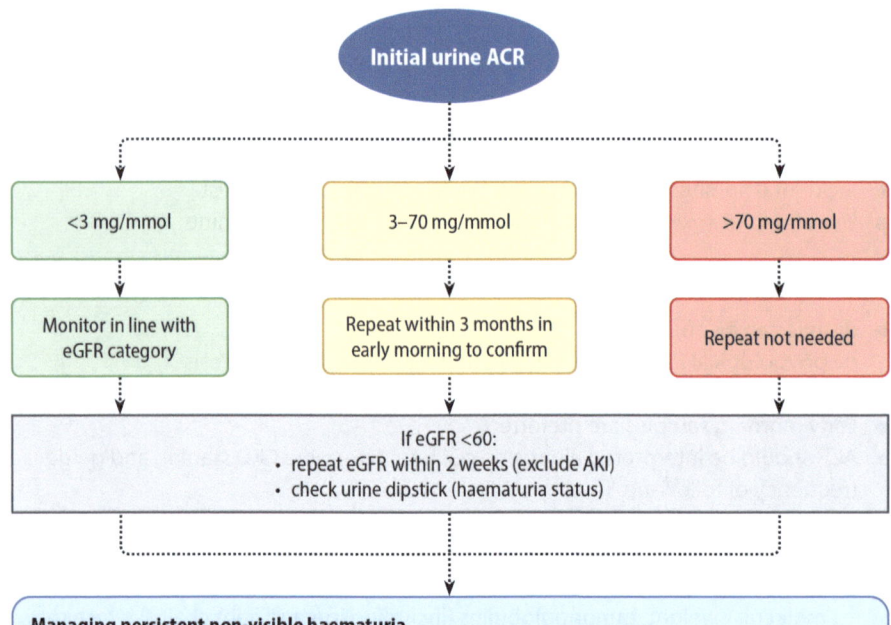

Adapted from: CKS NICE (revised 2024) *Chronic kidney disease*. https://cks.nice.org.uk/topics/chronic-kidney-disease/

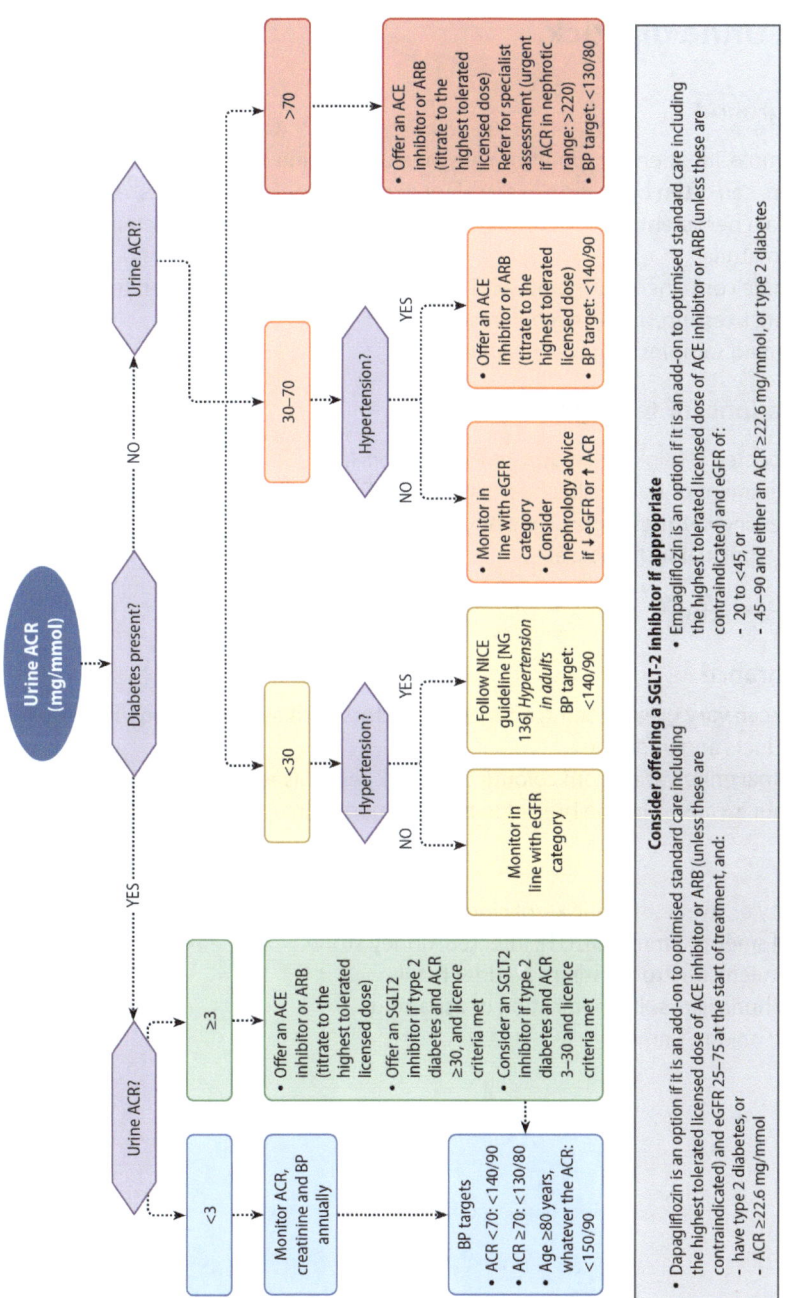

Adapted from: NICE (2021) Chronic kidney disease (G1-5, A1-3): managing proteinuria. www.nice.
org.uk/guidance/ng203/resources/visual-summary-chronic-kidney-disease-g15-a13-managing-proteinuria-
pdf-9206256495 and CKS NICE (revised 2024) *Chronic kidney disease.* https://cks.nice.org.uk/topics/chronic-
kidney-disease

1.7.2 Urine dipstick

Background

- A simple, inexpensive, point-of-care means of testing urine samples
- There can often be benign or transient explanations for the results, e.g. UTI, but certain persistent findings require further investigation, e.g. persistent non-visible haematuria
- Sample containers with boric acid preservative should not be used to perform urine dipstick testing, as it can affect results
- Morning samples are most reliable

Indications for testing

- Suspected UTI in certain groups (see *Section 4.1.5*)
- Assessment of non-visible haematuria (see *Section 1.7.1*)
- Assessing ketones for possible new-onset type 1 diabetes (in conjunction with fingerprick blood glucose)

Interpretation

Appearance

- This can vary greatly, being affected by factors such as foods, drugs, metabolic products and infections
- Normal urine varies from colourless to dark yellow (see Table opposite); the yellow colour is caused by the breakdown of haemoglobin

Odour

- Fruity or sweet: diabetic ketoacidosis
- Foul smell of ammonia: UTI, infected kidney stone
- Faeculent: gastrointestinal–bladder fistula
- Sulphuric-like: sulfa medication or asparagus
- Diet: onions, garlic

Urine examination

Appearance	Pathological causes	Medication causes	Food causes
Cloudy	Contamination with vaginal mucus or epithelial cells, phosphaturia, infection (pyuria), lipiduria, hyperoxaluria	–	Hyperuricosuria (diet high in purine-rich foods)
Foamy	Dehydration, frank proteinuria	–	–
Brown	Bile pigments, myoglobin	Levodopa, metronidazole, nitrofurantoin, senna	Fava (broad) beans
Brown/black	Bile pigments, melanin, methaemoglobin, myoglobulin, porphyria, stool from fistula	Levodopa, methyldopa, metronidazole, nitrofurantoin	Aloe, senna, fava beans, cascara (coffee cherry tea)
Green or blue	Pseudomonal UTI, biliverdin	Amitriptyline, cimetidine, indigo carmine (diagnostic agent), indomethacin, prochlorperazine	Asparagus (green)
Orange	Bile pigments	Rifampicin, sulfasalazine	Carrots
Red	Haematuria, haemoglobinuria, myoglobinuria, porphyria	Phenothiazines, phenytoin, senna, rifampicin	Beetroot, blackberries, rhubarb
Purple	Bacterial overgrowth in long-term indwelling catheters	–	–
Yellow	Concentrated urine (orange to gold in dehydration)	–	Carrots, cascara (coffee cherry tea)

Adapted from Simerville, J.A., Maxted, W.C. and Pahira, J.J. (2005) Urinalysis: a comprehensive review. *Am Fam Physician*, **71(6):** 1153–62 (erratum in: *Am Fam Physician*, (2006) **74(7):**c1096) and Devkota, B.P. (2022) *Urinalysis*. Medscape. https://emedicine.medscape.com/article/2074001-overview#a2

Interpreting urine dipstick tests

Test result	Normal range and notes	Causes	False positives	False negatives
Bilirubin	Normal: negative	Biliary obstruction, hepatic disease (conjugated bilirubin is water-soluble)	Phenazopyridine	Chlorpromazine, prolonged light exposure, selenium, vitamin C
Blood	Normal: negative Significant haematuria occurs at 1+ or above: trace levels should be considered negative	Glomerular disorders, hypercalciuria, hyperuricosuria, kidney stones, trauma, tubular disorders, tumour, UTI, drugs, e.g. NSAIDs, warfarin	Exercise, menses, haemoglobinuria, myoglobinuria	High urine specific gravity, vitamin C
Glucose	Normal: negative	Diabetes, pregnancy, SGLT2-i use (an expected effect)	Levodopa	High pH, high urine specific gravity, uric acid, vitamin C
Ketones	Normal: negative	Diabetes, ketogenic diet, pregnancy, starvation	High urine specific gravity, low pH	Delay in examination of urine
Leucocyte esterase	Normal: negative Presence suggests UTI	UTI, STI, inflammation process	Contamination	Antibiotics, high glucose, protein or urine specific gravity, vitamin C
Nitrites	Normal: negative Created by nitrate-reducing bacteria, their presence has a higher specificity than leucocyte esterase for detecting UTI	UTI	Contamination, dipstick exposure to air	High urine specific gravity, bacteria that do not reduce nitrates (Enterococcus), vitamin C, short bladder incubation time (<4 hours)

Test result	Normal range and notes	Causes	False positives	False negatives
pH	May vary from 4.5–8.0 (often 5.5–6.5 because of metabolic activity)	High: carbonic anhydrase inhibitors, heavy antacid use, potassium/sodium citrate use, high citrate diet, UTI (urease-positive bacteria such as *Proteus*), type I renal tubular acidosis, calcium phosphate and staghorn stones Low: diet, e.g. high protein, acid fruits (e.g. cranberries), uric acid and cystine stones	-	-
Protein	Dipstick tests detect many proteins but are most sensitive to albumin A protein finding of 1+ or greater suggests glomerular injury Dipstick testing that shows proteinuria should be followed by testing of U&E and urine ACR	Fever, glomerular disorders, tubular disorders, UTI	Concentrated or alkaline urine	Non-albumin proteinuria, acidic or diluted urine

Test result	Normal range and notes	Causes	False positives	False negatives
Urine specific gravity	Indicates hydration status: Near 1.010 suggests euvolaemia <1.003 is dilute >1.020 is concentrated Shows concentrations of dissolved substances in the urine (osmolality)	Low: adrenal insufficiency, aldosteronism, excessive fluid intake, renal failure, diabetes insipidus High: dehydration, glycosuria, SIADH	IV radio-opaque dyes, proteinuria	Alkaline urine, e.g. high-citrate diet
Urobilinogen	Normal: 0.1–1.0 mg/dL Urobilinogen is produced by the breakdown of bilirubin in the intestines	Intravascular haemolysis, hepatic disease (sometimes a normal finding)	Sulfonamides	Improper storage of sample, preservatives

Adapted from Simerville, J.A., Maxted, W.C. and Pahira, J.J. (2005) Urinalysis: a comprehensive review. *Am Fam Physician*, 71(6): 1153–62 (erratum in: *Am Fam Physician*, (2006) **74(7):** c1096) and Hitzeman, N., Greer, D. and Carpio, E. (2022) Office-based urinalysis: a comprehensive review. *Am Fam Physician*, **106(1):** 27–35B.

1.8 Endocrine

1.8.1 Thyroid function tests (TFT)

Adult reference ranges (Siemens):
Thyroid-stimulating hormone (TSH)	0.55–4.78 mU/L
Free T$_4$ (FT$_4$)	11.5–22.7 pmol/L
Free T$_3$ (FT$_3$)	3.5–6.54 pmol/L

Typical TFT result patterns in thyroid disease

Diagnosis	Test	
	TSH	FT$_3$/FT$_4$
Hyperthyroidism	↓	↑
Normal	↔	↔
Hypothyroidism	↑	↓

Atypical TFT result patterns and their causes

Test		Possible causes
TSH	FT$_3$/FT$_4$	
↓	↔	• Subclinical hyperthyroidism • Recent treatment for hyperthyroidism • Medications, e.g. steroids • Non-thyroidal illness
↑	↔	• Subclinical hypothyroidism • Poor concordance with thyroxine • Thyroxine malabsorption • Medications, e.g. amiodarone • Assay interference • Non-thyroidal illness recovery phase • TSH resistance
↔ or ↓	↓	• Non-thyroidal illness • Central hypothyroidism • Isolated TSH deficiency
↔ or ↑	↑	• Assay interference • Thyroxine replacement, including poor concordance • Medications, e.g. amiodarone • Non-thyroidal illness • TSH-secreting pituitary adenoma • Resistance to thyroid hormone • Disorders of thyroid hormone transport or metabolism

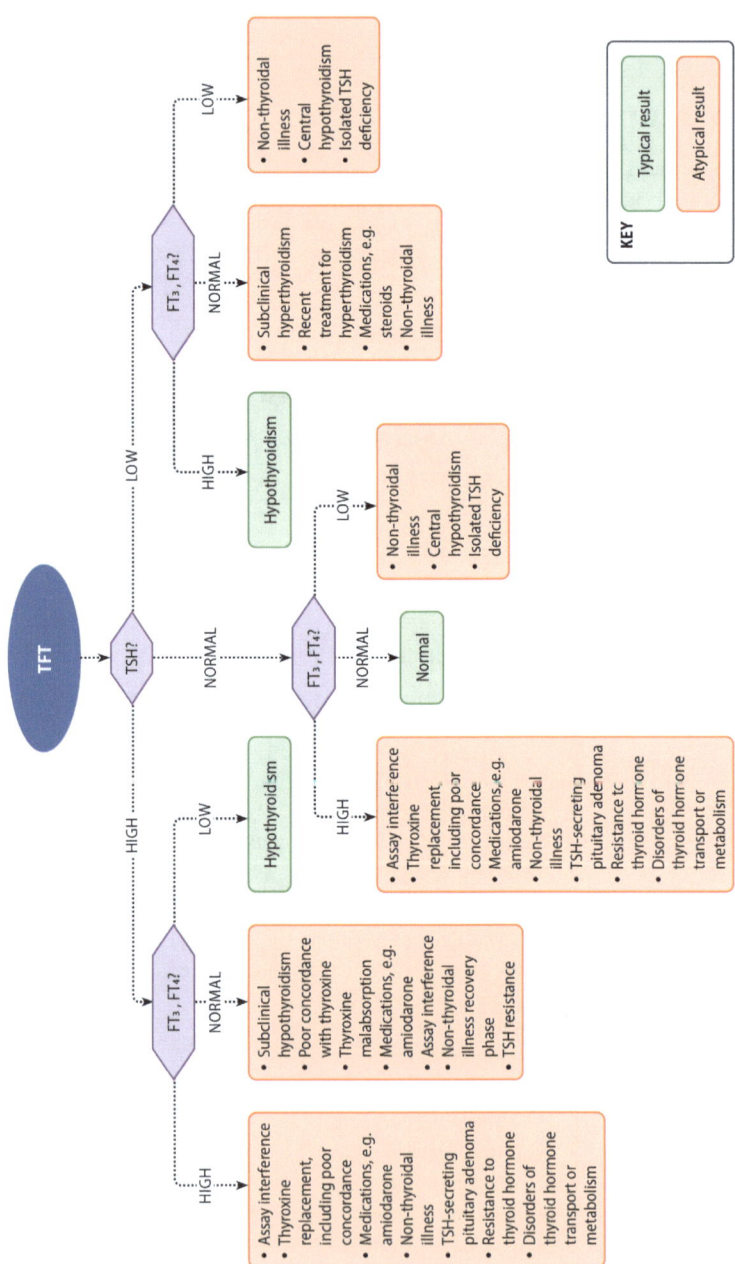

Adapted from Koulouri, O., Moran, C., Halsall, D., Chatterjee, K. and Gurnell, M. (2013) Pitfalls in the measurement and interpretation of thyroid function tests. *Best Pract Res Clin Endocrinol Metab*, **27(6)**: 745–62.

Background

- The first-line test is TSH or TSH and FT_4 (will vary between labs)
- FT_3 and thyroid autoantibodies may be reflexed by the laboratory as appropriate based on the TSH result, previous results, and available clinical details
- Disorders of thyroid function include overt and subclinical hypothyroidism and hyperthyroidism

Indications for testing

- Symptoms of hyper-/hypothyroidism
- Goitre
- Atrial fibrillation
- Dyslipidaemia
- Osteoporosis
- Subfertility, abnormal menstrual cycle, or miscarriage
- Type 1 diabetes
- Dementia
- Unexplained anxiety/depression
- Elderly or menopausal with non-specific symptoms
- Surveillance: annual check in:
  - o Down's syndrome
  - o Turner syndrome
  - o previous postpartum thyroiditis
  - o previous neck irradiation or surgery
  - o type 1 diabetes
  - o Addison's disease
  - o radioiodine or surgery for hyperthyroidism
- Drug monitoring
  - o amiodarone: baseline, then every 6 months, and up to 12 months after stopping
  - o lithium: baseline, then every 6–12 months
  - o antithyroid drugs (carbimazole, propylthiouracil): TFT tested every 1–3 months when initiating antithyroid drug therapy until stable, and annually if used as a long-term treatment
  - o thyroxine replacement in hypothyroidism: annual TSH only when stable

Interpretation

- Following treatment for hyperthyroidism, recovery of previously ↓ TSH can be delayed: FT_4 and FT_3 provide better information for clinical management
- TSH level can take up to 6 months to return to the reference range for people who had a very high TSH level before starting treatment with levothyroxine or a prolonged period of untreated hypothyroidism
- Non-adherence with thyroxine therapy: additional doses in the days before blood monitoring can produce ↑ TSH and ↑ FT_4
- Timing of blood tests: if thyroxine therapy is taken shortly before blood sampling, a ↑ TSH with normal or high-normal FT_4 may result

- Diurnal variation: the normal nocturnal peak in TSH may be delayed in night shift workers, those with irregular sleeping patterns, after vigorous exercise, and in mood disorders such as depression
- Non-thyroidal illness ('sick euthyroid syndrome'):
  - a wide range of acute or chronic non-thyroidal conditions, starvation and trauma can lead to abnormal TFTs which are not due to true dysfunction of the hypothalamic–pituitary–thyroid axis
  - TSH can be normal or ↓, then becomes ↑ during recovery from acute illness; FT_3/FT_4 can be normal, ↓ or ↑
  - TFTs should be delayed until 3 months post an acute illness
- Adrenal insufficiency: may be associated with ↑ TSH that reverses with glucocorticoid replacement
- Obesity: may ↑ TSH, which may falsely suggest subclinical hypothyroidism
- Age: mild TSH elevation may be a normal physiological adaption to ageing
- Drugs can affect the results, including:
  - supplements containing biotin and kelp
  - lithium, amiodarone, oestrogens, methadone, androgens, glucocorticoids, cholestyramine, iron salts, phenytoin, carbamazepine
  - excess thyroxine treatment
- Ethnicity: 3–4% of people of African origin have TSH levels below the reference range; levels may also be suppressed in the black non-Hispanic American population

Hyperthyroidism

Background

- Pathologically increased thyroid hormone production and secretion
- Overt hyperthyroidism: ↓ TSH, ↑ FT_3/FT_4
- Subclinical hyperthyroidism: ↓ TSH, FT_3/FT_4 ↔
- Secondary hyperthyroidism: TSH levels are inappropriately ↑ or ↔, but FT_3/FT_4 is ↑

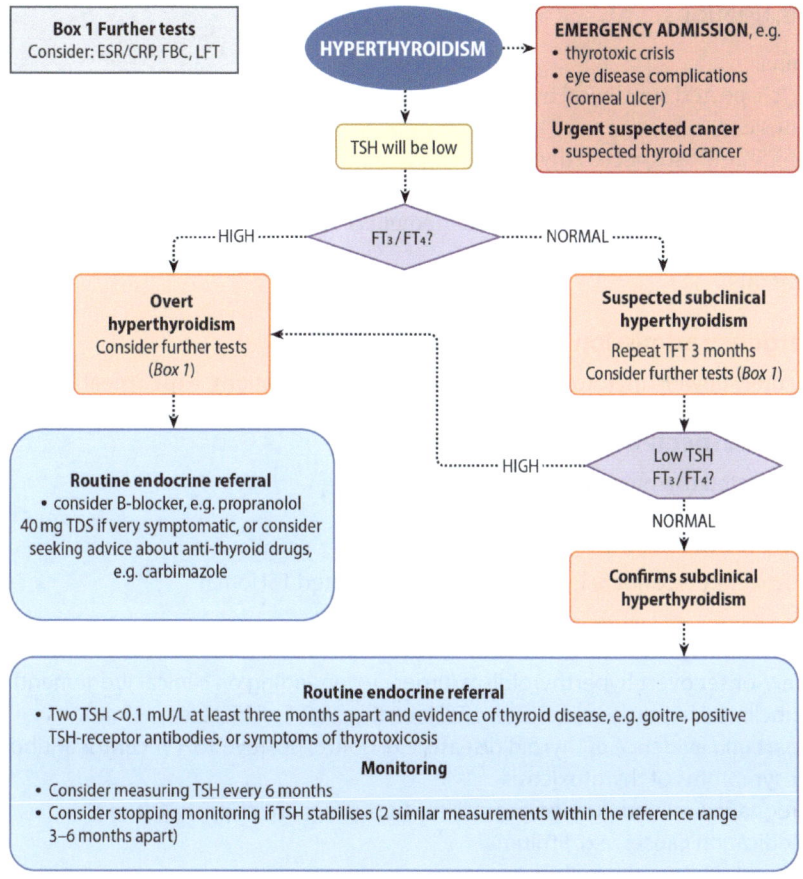

Box 1 Further tests
Consider: ESR/CRP, FBC, LFT

HYPERTHYROIDISM

EMERGENCY ADMISSION, e.g.
• thyrotoxic crisis
• eye disease complications (corneal ulcer)

Urgent suspected cancer
• suspected thyroid cancer

TSH will be low

FT₃/FT₄?

HIGH

NORMAL

Overt hyperthyroidism
Consider further tests
(*Box 1*)

Suspected subclinical hyperthyroidism
Repeat TFT 3 months
Consider further tests (*Box 1*)

Routine endocrine referral
• consider B-blocker, e.g. propranolol 40 mg TDS if very symptomatic, or consider seeking advice about anti-thyroid drugs, e.g. carbimazole

Low TSH
FT₃/FT₄?

HIGH

NORMAL

Confirms subclinical hyperthyroidism

Routine endocrine referral
• Two TSH <0.1 mU/L at least three months apart and evidence of thyroid disease, e.g. goitre, positive TSH-receptor antibodies, or symptoms of thyrotoxicosis
Monitoring
• Consider measuring TSH every 6 months
• Consider stopping monitoring if TSH stabilises (2 similar measurements within the reference range 3–6 months apart)

Adapted from NICE CKS (revised 2025) *Hyperthyroidism*. https://cks.nice.org.uk/topics/hyperthyroidism

Causes

- Primary: caused by abnormality of the thyroid gland, e.g. Graves' disease, toxic multinodular goitre, toxic thyroid nodule (adenoma); drugs (amiodarone, lithium)
- Secondary: pituitary adenoma 'TSHoma' (rare)

History and examination

- Symptoms: anxiety, palpitations, tremor, weight loss, diarrhoea and heat intolerance
- Signs: agitation, sinus tachycardia, goitre and/or thyroid nodules
- Graves' orbitopathy: excessive eye watering, double vision, change in visual acuity or colour vision, eyelid retraction or lid lag, proptosis
- Check: recent non-thyroidal illness, medications and risk factors for thyroid disease, e.g. smoking history, FHx thyroid disease, PMH autoimmune disease (type 1 diabetes)

Investigations

- Initial:
  - ○ suspected subclinical hyperthyroidism: repeat TFT 3 months after initial result
- Consider
  - ○ ESR/CRP: suspected thyroiditis
  - ○ FBC, LFT: for baseline if antithyroid drugs are to be started
  - ○ USS neck: palpable thyroid enlargement or focal nodularity

Referral

Emergency admission

- Acutely unwell (thyrotoxic crisis, eye disease complications, e.g. corneal ulcer)

Urgent suspected cancer

- Suspected thyroid malignancy

Urgent outpatient (endocrinology)

- Suspected secondary hyperthyroidism (suspected TSHoma)

Routine outpatient (endocrinology)

- New-onset overt hyperthyroidism (urgency depending on clinical judgement)
- Subclinical hyperthyroidism: two TSH readings <0.1 mU/L at least 3 months apart *and* evidence of thyroid disease, e.g. goitre, positive TSH-receptor antibodies, or symptoms of thyrotoxicosis
- Pregnancy-related queries: pre-conception, pregnant or postpartum
- Medication causes, e.g. lithium
- Graves' orbitopathy (ophthalmology)

Advice & Guidance (endocrinology)

- Treatment advice about antithyroid drugs, e.g. carbimazole
  - ○ initiation
  - ○ interpreting results to guide adjustments to therapy (if appropriate) and not under an endocrinology specialist
- Diagnostic uncertainty, e.g. atypical results

Hypothyroidism

Background

- Overt hypothyroidism: $\uparrow$ TSH (usually above 10 mU/L) and $\downarrow$ FT_3/FT_4
- Subclinical hypothyroidism: $\uparrow$ TSH, $FT_3/FT_4 \leftrightarrow$
- Secondary hypothyroidism: TSH levels are inappropriately $\downarrow$ or $\leftrightarrow$ (or rarely raised), but FT_3/FT_4 is $\downarrow$

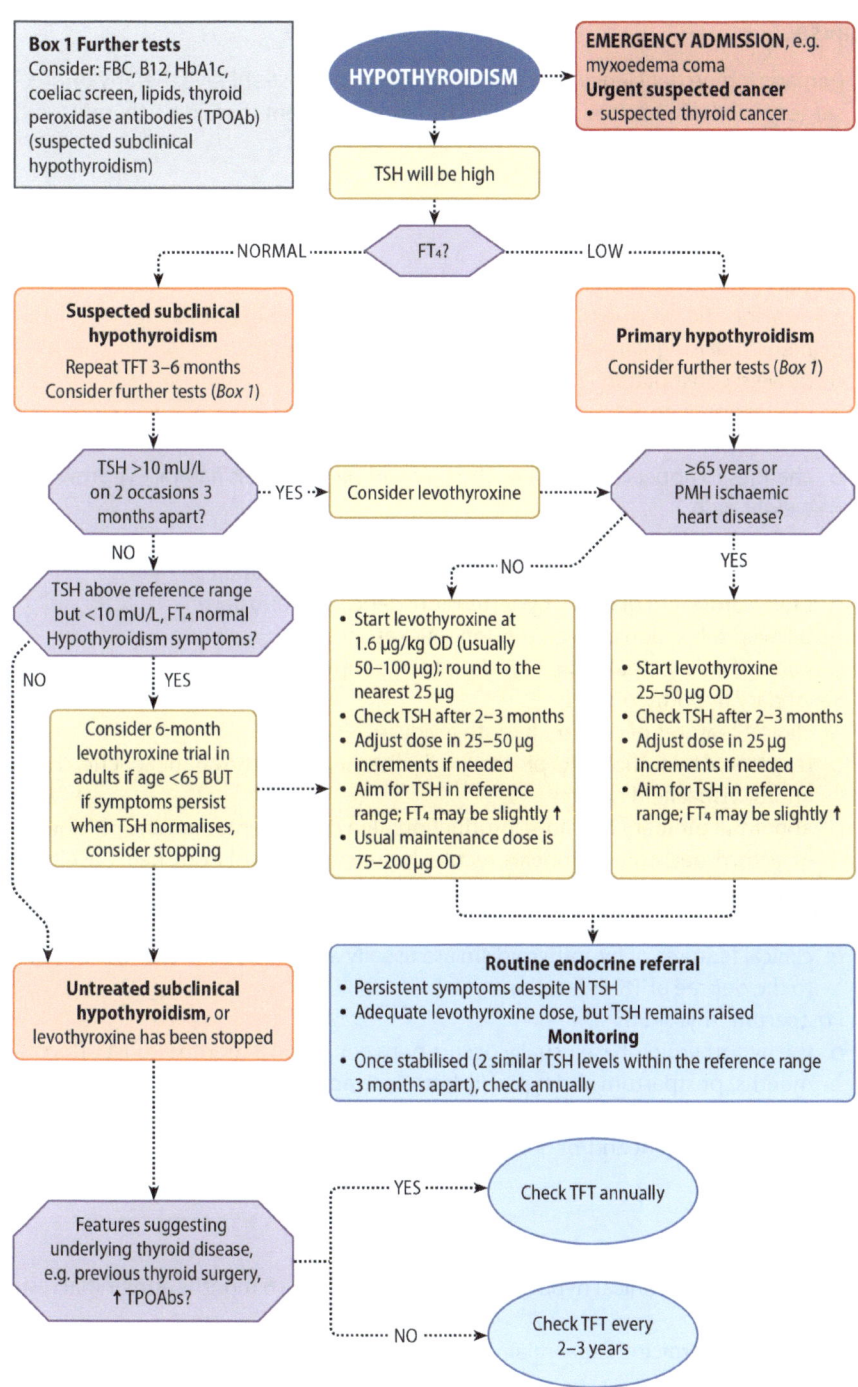

Box 1 Further tests
Consider: FBC, B12, HbA1c, coeliac screen, lipids, thyroid peroxidase antibodies (TPOAb) (suspected subclinical hypothyroidism)

HYPOTHYROIDISM

EMERGENCY ADMISSION, e.g. myxoedema coma
Urgent suspected cancer
- suspected thyroid cancer

TSH will be high

FT₄? ·····NORMAL····· ·····LOW·····

Suspected subclinical hypothyroidism
Repeat TFT 3–6 months
Consider further tests (*Box 1*)

Primary hypothyroidism
Consider further tests (*Box 1*)

TSH >10 mU/L on 2 occasions 3 months apart? ··· YES ··› Consider levothyroxine

≥65 years or PMH ischaemic heart disease?

NO

TSH above reference range but <10 mU/L, FT₄ normal Hypothyroidism symptoms?

NO   YES

Consider 6-month levothyroxine trial in adults if age <65 BUT if symptoms persist when TSH normalises, consider stopping

NO

YES

- Start levothyroxine at 1.6 µg/kg OD (usually 50–100 µg); round to the nearest 25 µg
- Check TSH after 2–3 months
- Adjust dose in 25–50 µg increments if needed
- Aim for TSH in reference range; FT₄ may be slightly ↑
- Usual maintenance dose is 75–200 µg OD

- Start levothyroxine 25–50 µg OD
- Check TSH after 2–3 months
- Adjust dose in 25 µg increments if needed
- Aim for TSH in reference range; FT₄ may be slightly ↑

Routine endocrine referral
- Persistent symptoms despite N TSH
- Adequate levothyroxine dose, but TSH remains raised
Monitoring
- Once stabilised (2 similar TSH levels within the reference range 3 months apart), check annually

Untreated subclinical hypothyroidism, or levothyroxine has been stopped

Features suggesting underlying thyroid disease, e.g. previous thyroid surgery, ↑ TPOAbs?

····· YES ·····› Check TFT annually

····· NO ·····› Check TFT every 2–3 years

Adapted from: NICE CKS (revised 2024) *Hypothyroidism*. https://cks.nice.org.uk/topics/hypothyroidism

Causes

- Primary: iodine deficiency, autoimmune thyroiditis, post-ablative therapy or surgery, medications (amiodarone and lithium), transient thyroiditis, thyroid infiltrative disorders
- Secondary: pituitary or hypothalamic disorder

History and examination

- Primary hypothyroidism
  - non-specific weakness, fatigue, arthralgia, myalgia, cold intolerance
  - menstrual irregularities; infertility or subfertility
  - bowels: constipation
  - depression, impaired concentration and memory
  - thyroid pain (in subacute thyroiditis)
  - changes to appearance: coarse dry hair and skin, hair loss (lateral eyebrows), weight gain
  - oedema, including swelling of the eyelids
  - hoarseness or deepening of the voice; goitre and/or nodules
  - bradycardia and diastolic hypertension; pericardial effusion
  - delayed relaxation of deep tendon reflexes
  - paraesthesia (carpal tunnel syndrome) or peripheral neuropathy
- Secondary hypothyroidism
  - clinical features of primary hypothyroidism
  - features of hypothalamic–pituitary axis disease, e.g. recurrent headache, diplopia and/or visual field defects
  - abnormal pituitary hormone production: skin depigmentation, atrophic breasts, galactorrhoea, amenorrhoea, erectile dysfunction, loss of body hair, Cushing's syndrome, or acromegaly
- Subclinical hypothyroidism
  - clinical features of hypothyroidism are usually absent, but if present, are related to the degree of TSH elevation
- Postpartum thyroiditis
  - the hypothyroid phase usually occurs between 3 and 8 months (most often at 6 months) postpartum and typically lasts 4–6 months
- Check: non-thyroidal illness, medications, FHx, associated autoimmune disease, thyroid enlargement and/or nodules

Investigations

- Initial:
  - suspected subclinical hypothyroidism: repeat TFT 3–6 months after initial result
- Consider
  - FBC, B12 (pernicious anaemia)
  - HbA1c, lipids
  - coeliac screen
  - thyroid peroxidase antibodies (TPOAb):

- subclinical hypothyroidism: ↑ can predict progression to overt hypothyroidism
  o USS neck: palpable thyroid enlargement or focal nodularity

Referral

Emergency admission

- Acutely unwell, e.g. myxoedema coma

Urgent suspected cancer

- Suspected thyroid malignancy

Urgent outpatient (endocrinology)

- Suspected secondary hypothyroidism
- Hypothyroidism with suspected adrenal insufficiency (urgency depending upon clinical judgement; do not start thyroid hormone replacement before specialist glucocorticoid replacement in suspected adrenal failure, as this can precipitate an adrenal crisis)

Routine outpatient (endocrinology)

- Pregnancy-related queries: pre-conception, pregnant or postpartum
- Medication causes, e.g. lithium

Advice & Guidance (endocrinology)

- Diagnostic uncertainty, e.g. atypical results
- Management advice, e.g. TSH not in normal range and/or ongoing symptoms despite >200 µg thyroxine and compliant with treatment, no other obvious cause

GP management tips

- Do **not** offer liothyronine (LT_3) or 'natural thyroid extracts'
- Thyroxine should be taken on an empty stomach in the morning before other food or medication

1.8.2 9am cortisol

No set cut-off for normal; see below

Background

- Random blood cortisol levels have limited use due to factors such as diurnal variation, effects of stress (very high levels >1000 nmol/L can be seen in acutely unwell patients or trauma) and oestrogen-containing preparations
- Blood samples for the initial cortisol level screen are best collected at 9am
- Secondary care confirm a suspected diagnosis of adrenal insufficiency using a short Synacthen test

- Seek endocrinology specialist advice before testing in people:
  - working shifts
  - taking long-term corticosteroids (should not be tested if taking higher than physiological doses i.e. ≥5 mg prednisolone or equivalent)
  - who have had IM or intra-articular steroids in the prior 6 weeks
  - receiving oral oestrogen treatment, e.g. oral contraceptive pill (OCP), hormone replacement therapy (HRT) (need to stop taking it for 6 weeks before testing)
  - who are pregnant

Indications for test

- Suspected adrenal insufficiency
  - **NB: if adrenal crisis is suspected (hypotension, hypovolaemic shock, acute abdominal pain, vomiting, and reduced level of consciousness), emergency admission should be arranged: emergency treatment should never be delayed for investigations**
  - possible presentations may include:
    - persistent, non-specific symptoms, e.g.
      - severe fatigue (seen in 94% of patients with adrenal insufficiency)
      - weakness (91%)
      - weight loss (86%)
      - hyper-pigmentation (80%)
      - dizziness/blackouts (79%)
      - reduced blood pressure (77%)
      - nausea (73%)
      - vomiting (55%)
      - difficulty concentrating (54%)
      - muscle/joint pains (52%)
      - salt cravings (51%)
      - headache (33%)
      - stomach pains (33%)
    - if symptoms worsen when thyroxine is started for hypothyroidism
    - type 1 diabetes with recurrent unexplained hypoglycaemic episodes
    - other autoimmune conditions, e.g. vitiligo, pernicious anaemia, chronic active hepatitis, alopecia and coeliac disease
    - ↓ sodium and ↑ potassium on blood biochemistry (**normal levels do not exclude the diagnosis**); other blood findings may include:
      - borderline or ↓ blood glucose
      - mild or moderate hypercalcaemia
      - anaemia, mild eosinophilia, and/or lymphocytosis
      - ↑ liver transaminases
      - ↑ TSH
- Hypopituitarism (secondary care testing)

Interpretation

Check local reference ranges, but as a guide:
- <100 nmol/L: emergency admission if high clinical suspicion of adrenal insufficiency
- 100–300 nmol/L: urgent endocrine referral for short Synacthen test
  - postural hypotension and/or electrolyte disturbance are indications for admission
- >300 nmol/L: adrenal insufficiency unlikely but consider endocrine referral if strong clinical suspicion persists

1.8.3 Parathyroid hormone (PTH)

Normal range 2.0–8.5 pmol/L (when the calcium is normal) (Siemens)

Background

- PTH is secreted by the parathyroid glands and plays an important role in calcium homeostasis; levels vary during the day
- Serum calcium regulates PTH via negative feedback: ↓ calcium stimulates ↑ PTH
- PTH causes:
  - ↑ calcium reabsorption by the kidneys
  - calcium and phosphate release from bone
  - ↑ calcium absorption from the gut via ↑ vitamin D production
- PTH should be tested with a simultaneous calcium level
- ↓ magnesium inhibits PTH

Indications for test

- Investigate abnormal calcium levels
  - distinguish between parathyroid and non-parathyroid causes
  - NICE suggests measure PTH if adjusted calcium is either:
    - ≥2.6 mmol/L on at least 2 separate occasions **or**
    - ≥2.5 mmol/L on at least 2 separate occasions and primary hyperparathyroidism is suspected
    - do not routinely repeat PTH measurement in primary care
- Monitoring patients with renal disease
- Assessing patients post parathyroidectomy or thyroidectomy (secondary care)

Interpretation

- PTH should be interpreted in conjunction with:
  - clinical presentation
  - serum calcium, magnesium, phosphate, creatinine and vitamin D levels
- Seek specialist advice if PTH is either:
  - above the midpoint of the reference range and primary hyperparathyroidism is suspected, or
  - below the midpoint of the reference range with a concurrent adjusted calcium ≥2.6 mmol/L

- Do not offer further investigations for primary hyperparathyroidism if PTH is:
  - within reference range but below the midpoint of the reference range and the adjusted calcium is <2.6 mmol/L
- Consider malignancy if PTH is below the lower limit of the reference range

Diagnosis	Background	PTH	Calcium	Phosphate
Primary hyper-parathyroidism	Most common type of hyperparathyroidism Caused by parathyroid gland issue: solitary parathyroid adenoma (85%), parathyroid hyperplasia (15%), parathyroid carcinoma (<1%) Can be difficult to differentiate from familial hypocalciuric hypercalcaemia, an inherited, lifelong benign condition	↑ (or inappropriately ↔)	↑	↔ or ↓
Secondary hyperpara-thyroidism	Appropriate ↑ PTH in response to ↓ calcium or ↑ phosphate Causes: chronic renal failure, vitamin D deficiency, malabsorption, medications, e.g. thiazide diuretics, lithium, phosphates, steroids, isoniazid, rifampicin If renal function normal, may be due to resistance to PTH action (pseudohypoparathyroidism)	↑	↓	↔ or ↑
Tertiary hyper-parathyroidism	Long-standing secondary hyperparathyroidism leads to autonomous hypersecretion of PTH (advanced renal failure)	↑	↑	↑
Paraneoplastic hypercalcaemia	Caused by parathyroid-related peptide	↓	↑	↓
Hypoparathy-roidism	Ensure magnesium is normal	↓ (or inappropriately ↔)	↓	↑

Adapted from Sell, J., Ramirez, S. and Partin, M. (2022) Parathyroid disorders. *Am Fam Physician*, **105(3):** 289–98, GPNotebook (reviewed 2024) *Parathyroid hormone (PTH) interpretation of PTH results.* https://gpnotebook.com/en-GB/pages/diabetes-and-endocrinology/parathyroid-hormone-pth-interpretation-of-pth-results and Insogna, K.L. (2018) Primary hyperparathyroidism. *N Engl J Med*, **37:** 1050–9.

1.8.4 Prolactin

Normal range (Siemens):
♀ <50 years: 59–619 mU/L
♀ ≥50 years: 38–430 mU/L
♂ ≥21 years: 45–375 mU/L

Background

- Prolactin is secreted by the anterior cells of the pituitary gland
- Essential for normal production of human breast milk
- Control of prolactin is through the suppressive effect of dopamine from the hypothalamus
- Concentrations vary over 24 hours, rising during sleep and peaking in the morning
- Ideally test at least 1 hour after waking and before eating, after resting for 30 minutes
- Macroprolactin is a protein-bound form of prolactin which is not biologically active, i.e. it is not pathological. Delayed clearance of macroprolactin may produce artificially ↑ prolactin levels. Samples with prolactin >700 mU/L are therefore reflex tested for the presence of macroprolactin
- Levels <700 mU/L are not likely to be clinically significant

Indications for test

- Determine the cause of galactorrhoea, e.g. prolactinoma
- Suspected pituitary tumour (prolactinoma)
- Female: assess infertility, oligomenorrhoea, amenorrhoea, galactorrhoea, hirsutism
- Male: assess hypogonadism (e.g. erectile dysfunction (ED), gynaecomastia) and infertility
- Evaluate pituitary gland function (along with other hormones), e.g. in hypopituitarism (secondary care assessment)

Interpretation

Causes of ↑ prolactin:
- Physiological
  - recent sleep
  - recent exercise
  - pregnancy
  - breastfeeding
  - stress: physical or psychological, e.g. surgery, venepuncture (can double or occasionally quadruple basal concentrations)
  - recent breast examination (test should be delayed for at least 48 hours)
- Intracranial
  - pituitary tumours, e.g. prolactinomas and other tumours
  - head injury
  - post-seizure

- Endocrine/metabolic
  - hypothyroidism
  - renal failure
  - liver cirrhosis
  - polycystic ovarian syndrome (PCOS)
- Drugs
  - dopamine receptor antagonists, e.g. domperidone, metoclopramide, phenothiazines, risperidone
  - antidepressants, e.g. tricyclic antidepressants (TCAs), SSRIs
  - verapamil
  - opiates
  - omeprazole
  - oestrogens

Causes of ↓ prolactin:

- hypopituitarism
- drugs, e.g. dopamine, levodopa, bromocriptine

GP management tips

- Medication-induced hyperprolactinaemia:
  - seek advice from prescribing clinician or endocrinology about medication dose changes and monitoring
  - <3000 mU/L: likely due to medications, repeat in 6–12 months to monitor
  - >3000 mU/L: routine referral (endocrinology) for further investigations
- <1000 mU/L:
  - rarely pathological and is likely due to stress of venepuncture
  - repeat after 4–6 weeks; consider routine referral (endocrinology) if remains abnormal, symptomatic or of unknown cause
- Levels >1000 mU/L
  - routine referral (endocrinology): usually warrants further investigation (e.g. pituitary MRI, visual field testing, anterior pituitary function testing)
  - urgent referral (endocrinology): if >5000 mU/L

1.9 Cardiovascular

1.9.1 Haemoglobin A1c (HbA1c)

Normal range <42 mmol/mol (IFCC traceable)

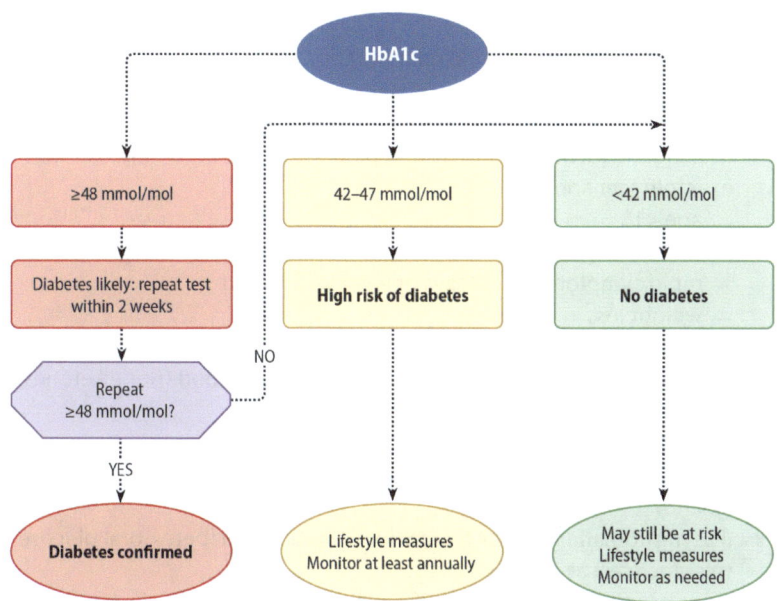

Adapted from Kilpatrick, E.S. and Atkin, S.L. (2014) Using haemoglobin A(1c) to diagnose type 2 diabetes or to identify people at high risk of diabetes. *BMJ*, **348:** g2867.

Background

- HbA1c measures the amount of glucose attached to haemoglobin and can be used to diagnose suspected diabetes; fasting is not required for the test
- Suspect diabetes if a person presents with persistent hyperglycaemia with or without symptoms. Persistent hyperglycaemia is defined as:
  - HbA1c ≥48 mmol/mol
  - fasting plasma glucose concentration ≥7.0 mmol/L
  - random plasma glucose ≥11.1 mmol/L in the presence of symptoms or signs of diabetes
- Diagnosis of diabetes:
  - do not use random plasma glucose as criterion
  - symptomatic: a single abnormal HbA1c or fasting plasma glucose level can be used
    - repeat testing is sensible to confirm the diagnosis
  - asymptomatic: do not diagnose diabetes based on a single abnormal HbA1c or plasma glucose result; arrange repeat testing with the **same test** to confirm the diagnosis
    - if the repeat test result is normal, monitor for the development of diabetes, the frequency depending on clinical judgement
  - NB: gestational diabetes is diagnosed using an oral glucose tolerance test (secondary care)

Indications for test

- Suspected type 2 diabetes (stable patient)
- **Do not use** HbA1c in the following groups:
  - ○ suspected type 1 diabetes
    - ■ use fingerprick blood glucose and point-of-care blood / urine ketones
    - ■ example scenarios:
      - – age <18
      - – acutely ill
      - – rapid symptom onset (days or weeks, <2 months)
      - – weight loss
  - ○ rapid-onset diabetes
    - ■ use fingerprick blood glucose and point-of-care blood / urine ketones
    - ■ example scenarios:
      - – steroid-induced diabetes
      - – post-pancreatitis or pancreatic surgery
  - ○ pregnancy
    - ■ if asymptomatic with risk factors for gestational diabetes, oral glucose tolerance test at 24–28 weeks
  - ○ may not be reliable in these specific comorbidities, thus use fasting blood glucose and point-of-care blood / urine ketones instead:
    - ■ iron and B12 deficiency
    - ■ recent blood transfusion (wait 6 months)
    - ■ renal dialysis
    - ■ haemoglobinopathies, thalassaemia
    - ■ ↓ red cell survival:
      - – haemolytic anaemia
      - – splenomegaly, post-splenectomy
      - – antiretroviral drugs

Interpretation

- HbA1c ≥48 mmol/mol: diabetes (repeat test within 2 weeks to confirm)
- HbA1c 42–47 mmol/mol: pre-diabetes
- HbA1c <42 mmol/mol: no diabetes

GP management tips

- Blood ketones: ketonaemia >3 mmol/L or >2+ ketonuria on strip testing with elevated random blood glucose is a medical emergency
- If unwell, patients should follow sick day rules

Blood ketones (mmol/L)	Action
<0.6	Normal
0.6–1.5	Slightly high: test again in 1–2 hours
1.6–3.0	At risk of DKA: assess and consider admission
>3	Likely DKA: call 999 or attend A&E

Adapted from www.nhs.uk/conditions/diabetic-ketoacidosis

- The table below provides a conversion guide between HbA1c (old and new units) and average blood glucose readings (UK and European / USA units)

HbA1c (%)	HbA1c (mmol/mol)	Average blood glucose UK (mmol/L)	Average blood glucose Europe and USA (mg/dL)
5	31	5.4	97
6	42	7.0	126
7	53	8.6	154
8	64	10.2	183
9	75	11.8	212
10	86	13.4	240
11	97	14.9	269
12	108	16.5	298

Adapted from Luthra, S., Viola, L., Navaratnarajah, M., Thirukumaran, D. and Velissaris, T. (2024) Glycated haemoglobin (HbA$_{1c}$) in cardiac surgery: a narrative review. *J Clin Med*, **14(1):** 23.

- Consider NICE guideline NG12 (*Suspected cancer: recognition and referral*), which recommends:
  - consider direct access USS in women aged ≥55 with visible haematuria and ↑ blood glucose levels (endometrial cancer)
  - consider urgent direct access CT scan (within 2 weeks), or an urgent USS if CT is not available, in patients aged ≥60 with new-onset diabetes and weight loss (pancreatic cancer)

1.9.2 Lipids

Adult ranges (Siemens)
Total cholesterol – interpret within clinical context
Triglycerides <2.0 mmol/L
HDL-cholesterol ♂ >1.0 mmol/L, ♀ >1.2 mmol/L
Non-HDL-cholesterol – interpret within clinical context
LDL-cholesterol – interpret within clinical context
Total cholesterol to HDL ratio – interpret using QRISK3 or other risk calculator

Background

- Dyslipidaemia is an established risk factor for CVD and can be modified by lifestyle changes and lipid-lowering treatment
- A full lipid profile involves taking a non-fasting blood sample to measure:
  - total cholesterol, high-density lipoprotein cholesterol (HDL-C) and triglyceride (TG) levels
  - low-density lipoprotein cholesterol (LDL-C) and non-HDL cholesterol (the difference between total and HDL cholesterol) are then calculated
  - fasting is not required
- Interpretation of the lipid result will involve checking:
  - the indication for testing (general health check, medication monitoring)
  - any current therapies for lipid management
  - relevant comorbidities
- Exclude and address secondary hypercholesterolaemia, rechecking lipids (if possible) after the condition has resolved or the medication stopped, e.g.
  - endocrine: diabetes, hypothyroidism, Cushing's
  - liver disease: cholestatic, e.g. primary biliary cholangitis (PBC)
  - renal: nephrotic syndrome, end-stage kidney disease
  - infection: HIV
  - other: anorexia nervosa, pregnancy, alcohol excess, obesity, monoclonal gammopathy of undetermined significance (MGUS)
  - medications: androgens, ciclosporin, thiazide diuretics, corticosteroids, retinoic acid derivatives, β-blockers and antiretroviral therapy

NICE vs. European guidelines

- UK clinicians will be most familiar with NICE guidance on managing lipids
- However, the European guidelines by the European Society of Cardiology and European Atherosclerosis Society (ESC/EAS) introduce some important considerations, including stricter targets; follow your local lipid management pathway

Comparison of NICE vs. ESC/EAS guidelines

NICE	ESC/EAS
Assessing risk	
QRISK3 is used to calculate the estimated CVD risk within the next 10 years for those aged 25–84 without CVD, but including type 2 diabetes Consider using a lifetime risk tool, such as QRISK3-lifetime, for people with a 10-year QRISK3 score <10% and people aged <40 who have CVD risk factors Do not use a risk assessment tool in those at high risk of CVD: • aged ≥85 • type 1 diabetes • eGFR <60 and/or albuminuria • FH • pre-existing CVD	ESC/EAS risk charts estimate 10-year risk of CVD death
Risk stratification	
Management is based on categories of primary or secondary prevention Primary prevention includes people with: • QRISK3 ≥10%, including those with type 2 diabetes • type 1 diabetes, CKD, or FH (or other inherited disorders of lipid metabolism) • Aged ≥85 Secondary prevention includes people with established CVD	People are categorised according to CV risk levels, e.g. **Very high** • History of CVD • Diabetes with: o target organ damage, or o at least 3 major risk factors, or o type 1 diabetes for >20 years • Severe CKD (eGFR <30) • FH with CVD or another major risk factor **High** • Markedly elevated single risk factors: o TC >8 mmol/L o LDL-C >4.9 mmol/L o BP ≥180/110 mmHg • FH without other major risk factors • Diabetes without target organ damage • Moderate CKD (eGFR 30–59) **Moderate** • Young patients (type 1 diabetes <35 years; type 2 <50 years) with duration <10 years, without other risk factors **Low** Calculated SCORE <1% for 10-year risk of fatal CVD

Comparison of NICE vs. ESC/EAS guidelines	
NICE	**ESC/EAS**
Treatment targets	
Primary prevention: • >40% reduction in non-HDL levels Secondary prevention: • LDL ≤2.0 mmol/L *or* • non-HDL ≤2.6 mmol/L	Tighter targets compared to NICE **Very high** Primary or secondary prevention: • ≥50% LDL-C reduction from baseline, and • LDL-C <1.4 mmol/L **High** • ≥50% LDL-C reduction from baseline, and • LDL-C <1.8 mmol/L **Moderate** • LDL-C <2.6 mmol/L **Low** • LDL-C <3.0 mmol/L

Indications for test

● Assessment in primary prevention of CVD
● Monitoring therapy in primary and secondary prevention of CVD
● Suspected familial hypercholesterolaemia (FH)

Interpretation

Primary prevention

● Offer lifestyle advice
● If lifestyle change alone is ineffective or inappropriate, e.g. thought to be at higher CVD risk due to comorbidities or clinical judgement, offer statin therapy for adults who have any of the following:
  ○ age ≤84 and QRISK ≥10%, including type 2 diabetes
  ○ type 1 diabetes, if they have one or more of: age >40, diabetes for >10 years, established nephropathy, other CVD risk factors
  ○ eGFR <60 and/or albuminuria
  ○ FH
● Consider offering statin in the following:
  ○ age >85
  ○ age 18–40 with type 1 diabetes, including those with diabetes for ≤10 years
● If QRISK3 <10%, do not rule out statin treatment: consider patient preference and if other factors are present that may lead to risk being underestimated in certain groups:
  ○ treated for HIV
  ○ already taking medicines to treat CVD risk factors
  ○ recently stopped smoking

- o taking medicines that can cause dyslipidaemia, e.g. immunosuppressant drugs
- o with severe mental illness (schizophrenia, bipolar disorder or other psychoses)
- o with autoimmune or other systemic inflammatory disorders
- Treatment options, e.g.:
  - o first-line: high-intensity statin, e.g. atorvastatin 20 mg, increasing to maximum tolerated dose if needed to achieve targets
  - o combination treatment, e.g. statin and ezetimibe: if targets not achieved
  - o ezetimibe alone: if statin contraindicated or intolerance
  - o ezetimibe and bempedoic acid: if targets not achieved
  - o review every 3 months until target achieved, then monitor yearly
- Treatment target:
  - o NICE: >40% reduction in non-HDL levels
  - o ESC/EAS:
    - ▪ very high risk: ≥50% LDL-C reduction from baseline, and LDL-C <1.4 mmol/L
    - ▪ high risk: ≥50% LDL-C reduction from baseline and LDL-C <1.8 mmol/L
    - ▪ moderate risk: LDL-C <2.6 mmol/L
    - ▪ low risk: LDL-C <3.0 mmol/L
- Referral (routine lipid clinic):
  - o medication intolerance
  - o suspected FH / other inherited dyslipidaemia or extensive FHx of early CVD
  - o advice on indication for lipid-lowering treatment if unclear from initial assessment

Secondary prevention

- Treatment options, e.g.:
  - o first-line: offer high-intensity statin, e.g. atorvastatin 80 mg. Offer lower dose if:
    - ▪ CKD eGFR <60: offer atorvastatin 20 mg
    - ▪ medication interactions
    - ▪ increased risk of side-effects
    - ▪ patient request
  - o ezetimibe alone: if statin contraindicated or intolerance
  - o combination treatment, e.g. statin and ezetimibe: if targets not achieved
  - o review every 3 months until target achieved, then monitor yearly
- Treatment target:
  - o NICE: LDL-C ≤2.0 mmol/L or non-HDL ≤2.6 mmol/L
  - o ESC/EAS: ≥50% LDL-C reduction from baseline and LDL-C <1.4 mmol/L
- Referral (routine lipid clinic):
  - o LDL-cholesterol persistently >2.6 mmol/L despite maximum tolerated therapy

Triglycerides (TG)

Background

- Routinely measured as part of a full lipid profile to enable LDL calculation
- May be ↑ on a non-fasting sample due to dietary TG; consider fasting sample

- May be due to primary causes, e.g. inherited conditions (familial combined hyperlipidaemia)
- Exclude common secondary causes: alcohol excess, obesity, diabetes, hypothyroidism, and medications, e.g. steroids, oral oestrogen therapy, β-blockers, oral retinoids
- CVD risk may be underestimated by risk assessment tools
- Optimise other CVD risk factors
- There are no UK guidelines stating TG treatment targets

Management

- NICE does not provide specific primary care treatment advice and targets:
  - TG >20 mmol/L and not due to excess alcohol or poor glycaemic control: urgent specialist review
  - TG 10–20 mmol/L:
    - repeat fasting TG after 5 days, but within 2 weeks, *and*
    - review for secondary causes, *and*
    - seek specialist advice if TG remains >10 mmol/L
  - TG 4.5–9.9 mmol/L:
    - be aware of CVD risk underestimation by risk assessment tools, *and*
    - optimise other CVD risk factors present, *and*
    - seek specialist advice if non-HDL-C >7.5 mmol/L
- ESC advises:
  - CVD risk increases when fasting TG >1.7 mmol/L, but medications to lower TG are advised only in the following groups:
    - high-risk patients when TG >2.3 mmol/L and cannot be lowered by lifestyle measures
      - first-line: statins
      - second-line: add fenofibrate or bezafibrate with statins
    - in primary prevention, those who are at LDL-C goal with TG >2.3 mmol/L:
      - consider fenofibrate or bezafibrate in combination with statins
- Referral:
  - emergency admission:
    - symptoms of pancreatitis
  - urgent (lipid clinic):
    - unexplained TG >20 mmol/L
  - routine (lipid clinic):
    - unexplained TG >10 mmol/L
    - TG 4.5–9.9 mmol/L and non-HDL-C >7.5 mmol/L
    - management advice if targets not attained on maximum tolerated therapy
      - NICE recommends icosapent ethyl as an option for reducing the risk of CV events in adults
        - taking statins
        - who have a high risk of CV events

   ☐ have raised fasting TG ≥1.7 mmol/L
   ☐ established CVD, e.g. history of MI or unstable angina requiring hospitalisation, coronary or other arterial revascularisation procedures, coronary heart disease, ischaemic stroke or peripheral arterial disease (PAD)
   ☐ LDL-C >1.04 mmol/L and ≤2.60 mmol/L

Familial hypercholesterolaemia (FH)

Background

- An inherited condition characterised by a high serum cholesterol concentration present from birth
- Assess previous results: the criteria below would not apply if the prior cholesterol levels have been below the stated thresholds for years
- Suspect FH in adults with:
  - total cholesterol >7.5 mmol/L *and/or*
  - a personal history or FHx of premature coronary heart disease (an event before 60 years in an index person or first-degree relative (parent, sibling, child))
- Although many people have raised cholesterol due to polygenic and lifestyle factors, the likelihood of having heterozygous FH increases with total cholesterol >7.5 mmol/L; an untreated LDL cholesterol >10 mmol/L may be suggestive of homozygous FH
- In primary care, consider systematic record searches for people at highest risk of FH, including people:
  - age <30 years with a total cholesterol >7.5 mmol/L *and those*
  - age ≥30 years with a total cholesterol >9.0 mmol/L
- If FH is suspected:
  - check two measurements of LDL cholesterol
    - consider a clinical diagnosis of homozygous FH in adults with LDL cholesterol >13 mmol/L
  - assess for clinical signs of FH, e.g. tendon xanthomata, eyelid xanthelasma, or corneal arcus; the absence of signs does not exclude a diagnosis of FH
  - exclude and address secondary hypercholesterolaemia: recheck lipids (if possible) after the condition has resolved or the drug reviewed
    - endocrine: diabetes, hypothyroidism, Cushing's
    - liver disease: cholestatic, e.g. PBC
    - renal: nephrotic syndrome, end-stage kidney disease
    - infection: HIV
    - other: anorexia nervosa, pregnancy, alcohol excess, obesity, MGUS
    - medications: androgens, ciclosporin, thiazide diuretics, corticosteroids, retinoic acid derivatives, β-blockers, and anti-retroviral therapy
- Use the Simon Broome criteria to aid clinical diagnosis of FH in primary care

Simon Broome criteria (adult)	
Definite FH	**Possible FH**
Total cholesterol >7.5 mmol/L and/or LDL-C >4.9 mmol/L	
and	
Tendon xanthomata in the patient, a 1st-degree (parent, sibling, or child) or a 2nd-degree relative (grandparent, uncle or aunt)	FHx of myocardial infarction in a 1st-degree relative aged <60 or in 2nd-degree relative aged <50
or	
DNA-based evidence of an LDL-receptor mutation, familial defective apo B-100, or a *PCSK9* mutation (likely unknown in primary care setting)	FHx of raised total cholesterol >7.5 mmol/L in adult 1st- or 2nd-degree relative or >6.7 mmol/L in child or sibling (of the person with suspected FH) aged <16 years

Management

- Make a clinical diagnosis of FH in people who meet the Simon Broome criteria for 'possible' or 'definite' FH
- Do not use QRISK tool to decide upon treatment
- Treatment options, e.g.:
  - first-line: high-intensity statin
  - ezetimibe alone: if statin contraindicated
  - combination treatment, e.g. statin and ezetimibe: if targets not achieved
- Treatment target:
  - NICE:
    - heterozygous FH: >50% reduction in baseline LDL-C
    - homozygous FH: to be managed by lipid clinic
  - ESC:
    - very high risk of CVD:
      - ≥50% reduction in baseline LDL-C and LDL-C <1.4 mmol/L
    - in the absence of CVD or another major risk factor, patients with FH are categorised as high risk:
      - ≥50% reduction in baseline LDL-C and LDL-C <1.8 mmol/L
- Referral:
  - routine (lipid clinic):
    - all people with a clinical diagnosis of definite or possible FH for confirmation of the diagnosis and initiation of cascade testing, **but do not wait to treat**
    - people with cholesterol level >9.0 mmol/L or a non-HDL-C >7.5 mmol/L, even in the absence of a first-degree FHx of premature coronary heart disease (NICE)
    - management advice if targets not attained on maximum tolerated therapy

Lipoprotein(a) (Lp(a))

Background

- Check local pathways and availability
- Lp(a) is established as a risk factor for CVD and calcific aortic valve stenosis, with levels being genetically determined
- Serum lipoprotein(a) levels should be measured in those with:
  - a PMH or FHx of premature CVD (<60 years of age)
  - first-degree relatives with high Lp(a) levels (>200 nmol/L)
  - FH or other genetic dyslipidaemias
  - calcific aortic valve stenosis
  - a borderline increased (but <15%) 10-year risk of a cardiovascular (CV) event
- Levels need only be measured once, unless a secondary cause is suspected, or for monitoring if a specific treatment is used (secondary care)

Interpretation

- The risk level is determined by the Lp(a) concentration:
  - minor: 32–90 nmol/L
  - moderate: 90–200 nmol/L
  - high   200–400 nmol/L
  - very high   >400 nmol/L

Management

- Raised levels need to be considered in light of the whole clinical picture, e.g. FHx, patient age, other CV risk factors
  - immediate treatment is not always indicated, but where necessary, the aim is to reduce CV risk by controlling hyperlipidaemia and other risk factors
  - treatment with moderate- or high-intensity statins may be needed
  - target LDL-C/non-HDL-C will depend on Lp(a) concentration and patient's overall CV risk
- Referral (routine lipid clinic):
  - Management advice if indication for treatment is unclear

1.9.3 N-terminal pro-B-type natriuretic peptide (NT-pro-BNP)

Threshold for referral >400 ng/L

Background

- Natriuretic peptides are released by the myocardium in response to pressure or fluid overload; levels are raised in people with heart failure
- There are several other causes of ↓ or ↑ NT-pro-BNP (see below)

- Testing can aid diagnostic decision-making in suspected heart failure; guidelines recommend referral for cardiac imaging and specialist assessment depending on the level
- There are two types available: B-type NP (BNP) and NT-pro-BNP; BNP is biologically active and has a shorter half-life, making it less stable; use what is available in your area
- The European Society of Cardiology (ESC) and NICE recommend testing in acute and chronic heart failure (HF), but the thresholds differ significantly in chronic HF:
  - ESC referral threshold: BNP ≥35 pg/mL or NT-pro-BNP ≥125 pg/mL
  - NICE referral threshold: BNP ≥100 pg/mL or NT-pro-BNP ≥400 pg/mL
- NB: it does not differentiate between heart failure with reduced ejection fraction, mildly reduced ejection fraction, and preserved ejection fraction
- Causes of ↑ NT-pro-BNP:
  - age >70
  - cardiac: left ventricular hypertrophy, myocardial ischaemia, tachycardia, right ventricular overload
  - pulmonary: pulmonary hypertension, pulmonary embolism (PE), chronic obstructive pulmonary disease (COPD), hypoxia
  - chronic disease: eGFR <60, diabetes, liver cirrhosis
  - sepsis
- Causes of ↓ NT-pro-BNP:
  - BMI >35
  - medications, e.g. diuretics, ACEi, ARBs, β-blockers, spironolactone
  - African–Caribbean family origin

Indications for test

- Suspected chronic heart failure

Interpretation

- <400 ng/L (47 pmol/L) in an untreated person
  - diagnosis of heart failure less likely
  - consider discussion with cardiology if clinical suspicion persists
- 400–2000 ng/L (47–236 pmol/L)
  - heart failure cannot be excluded
  - refer to cardiology for ECHO to be seen within 6 weeks
- >2000 ng/L (236 pmol/L)
  - urgent referral (cardiology) for ECHO to be seen in 2 weeks

1.10 Liver screen

1.10.1 Alpha-1 antitrypsin

Normal range 0.78–2.00 g/L

Background

- Alpha-1 antitrypsin (AAT) deficiency is a genetic disorder with an autosomal inheritance pattern: one allele is inherited from each parent and each allele is expressed equally
- Allele mutations cause ineffective activity of AAT, an enzyme responsible for neutralising neutrophil elastase
- Pulmonary and hepatic disease manifestations include emphysema, COPD, bronchiectasis and cirrhosis
- AAT is an acute phase reactant: be aware that levels may be falsely normal if there is inflammation
- Disease may still be present with borderline or even normal AAT levels

Indications for test

- Abnormal liver function tests screen: consider checking for AAT deficiency if there is a positive FHx (first-degree relative) or associated respiratory symptoms
  - o be aware that liver involvement is rare in adults

Interpretation

- If AAT level is low, the lab will reflex biochemical phenotyping
- Follow the advice of lab comments
- All individuals have two AAT alleles; it is the expression of both alleles that contributes to the phenotypic variance and severity
- Each allele, normal or abnormal, has a letter designation between A and Z
- The normal allele is designated 'M', so two normal copies would be MM
- An example of a carrier phenotype is PI*MZ
- An example of a patient with AAT deficiency is PI*ZZ
- Given the large number of possible alleles, there are hundreds of possible genotypes and phenotypes
  - o the Z allele is most widely associated with clinical AAT deficiency
  - o the S allele is a common variant that results in decreased functional AAT expression, although not as severe as with the Z allele

Phenotype interpretation		
Result	**Risk of liver disease**	**Interpretation**
MM	None	Normal Nil further action
MS	No increase	Carrier Unlikely to impact health
SS	No increase	Partial deficiency Unlikely to impact health
MZ	Slight increase	Carrier Unlikely to impact health
SZ	Slight increase	Affected Increased risk of COPD (but lower than in ZZ)
ZZ	High	Affected Significantly increased risk of COPD and liver disease; refer to respiratory and hepatology

Adapted from *Alpha-1 Antitrypsin Deficiency (AATD)*. www.newcastle-hospitals.nhs.uk/services/clinical-genetics-service/information-for-healthcare-professionals/routine-referrals/alpha-1-antitrypsin-deficiency-aatd and Camelier, A.A., Winter, D.H., Jardim, J.R. *et al.* (2008) Deficiência de alfa-1 antitripsina: diagnóstico e tratamento [Alpha-1 antitrypsin deficiency: diagnosis and treatment]. *J Bras Pneumol*, **34(7)**: 514–27.

GP management tips

- MM is normal and requires no further action
- For all other results:
  - consider genetic testing for partner if couple have children / are planning family
  - couples who are both identified as carriers: consider referral to genetics
  - refer hepatology: diagnostic uncertainty, management advice (especially ZZ)
  - offer lifestyle advice, e.g. smoking and alcohol

1.10.2 Caeruloplasmin

Normal range: 0.20–0.60 g/L (Siemens)
<0.10 g/L: highly suggestive of Wilson's disease (no absolute cut-off for diagnosis)

Background

- Caeruloplasmin is the major protein-bound form of copper and is an acute phase protein
- Many factors can cause ↑ or ↓ levels:

- o ↓ levels: Wilson's disease, malnutrition, malabsorption, and nephrotic syndrome
- o ↑ levels: infection, inflammation, malignancy, pregnancy, medications (e.g. oestrogen-containing medications, anti-epileptics, such as valproate)
- For many patients, a combination of tests reflecting disturbed copper metabolism may be needed as no single test is specific

Indications for test

- Abnormal liver function tests screen: consider checking for Wilson's disease if age <40

Interpretation

Refer hepatology if diagnostic uncertainty
- >0.32 g/L: Likely due to infection/inflammation
- 0.20–0.32 g/L: Wilson's disease is highly unlikely
- 0.10–0.19 g/L: Wilson's disease is not excluded
- <0.10 g/L: Highly suggestive of Wilson's disease; refer

1.11 Men's health

1.11.1 Male hormone profile

Normal adult ranges (Siemens)		
Follicle-stimulating hormone (FSH):	1.4–18.1 IU/L	
Luteinising hormone (LH):	<70 years:	1.5–9.3 IU/L
	≥70 years:	3.1–34.6 IU/L
Total testosterone (TT):	<50 years:	6.9–23.2 nmol/L
	≥50 years:	6.5–23.7 nmol/L
Sex hormone-binding globulin (SHBG):		
	<50 years:	12–54 nmol/L
	≥50 years:	17–72 nmol/L

Background

- Synthesis and release of the pituitary hormones FSH and LH is under the control of gonadotrophin-releasing hormone (GnRH) from the hypothalamus, and modulated by circulating gonadal steroids, e.g. testosterone
- FSH and LH can be used to assess the hypothalamo–pituitary–gonadal axis, often in conjunction with testosterone and prolactin

Indication for test

- Testosterone deficiency screening in men with consistent and multiple signs of testosterone deficiency, e.g. low sexual desire (even without a sexual partner), hair loss, changes in fat distribution, voice changes, infertility

- Erectile dysfunction and loss of early morning erections
- Suspected pituitary gland disorders, e.g. tumours (secondary care testing)
- Delayed puberty (secondary care testing)

Interpretation

Testosterone

- Secretion has diurnal variation and is suppressed post-prandially, so check fasting serum total testosterone between 7am and 11am
- If the serum testosterone level is low or borderline, arrange a repeat check preferably 4 weeks apart
  - o also check FSH, LH, SHBG and prolactin
- Check local referral pathways for guidance on the interpretation of testosterone levels
  - o refer to endocrine if levels are below the normal reference range

Follicle-stimulating hormone (FSH) and luteinising hormone (LH)

- Diagnosing male hypogonadism

Diagnosis	Notes	Testosterone	FSH/LH
Primary hypogonadism	Caused by intrinsic testicular dysfunction	↓	↑
Secondary (central) hypogonadism	Caused by impaired hypothalamo–pituitary function; likely to need full pituitary hormone profile NB: may be indistinguishable from that of non-gonadal illness, where there is physiological suppression of FSH/LH, e.g. due to obesity and type 2 diabetes that resolves upon recovery	↓	↓ or ↔

Sex hormone-binding globulin (SHBG)

- 60–70% of circulating testosterone is bound to SHBG
- SHBG-bound testosterone is biologically inactive compared to its unbound 'free' form
- In males with abnormal SHBG levels, total testosterone may give a misleading measure

- SHBG should be checked in men with an equivocal or borderline total testosterone, and can be used to calculate the serum free testosterone, which is generally more accurate; the lab can also provide a free androgen index value
- Causes of ↓ SHBG (and ↑ active testosterone):
  - insulin resistance
  - obesity
  - hyperprolactinaemia
  - hypothyroidism
- Causes of ↑ SHBG (and ↓ active testosterone):
  - hyperthyroidism
  - excess alcohol
  - liver disease
  - anticonvulsants

1.11.2 Prostate-specific antigen (PSA)

Normal range: age-specific cut-offs; see below

Background

- Protein produced by the prostate gland
- May be increased in prostate cancer, benign prostatic enlargement, prostatitis, UTI; it also increases naturally with age
- Counsel patients about the risks and benefits of the test
  - refer as urgent suspected cancer (urology) if the prostate feels malignant on digital rectal examination, regardless of the PSA level

Indications for test

- Considered in men with suspected prostate cancer
- Offered to men age >50 who request a PSA test

Interpretation

- Before a PSA test, people should not have:
  - an active UTI or within the previous 6 weeks
  - ejaculated in the previous 48 hours
  - exercised vigorously, e.g. cycling, in the previous 48 hours
  - had a urological intervention such as prostate biopsy in previous 6 weeks
- Consider urgent suspected cancer referral (urology) if PSA is above the threshold for their age (considering the person's preferences and any comorbidities)

Age-specific PSA ranges	
Age (years)	**PSA threshold (µg/L)**
<40	Use clinical judgement
40–49	>2.5
50–59	>3.5
60–69	>4.5
70–79	>6.5
>79	Use clinical judgement

Taken from NICE CKS (revised 2024) *Prostate cancer*. https://cks.nice.org.uk/topics/prostate-cancer

1.12 Women's health

1.12.1 Female hormone profile

Normal ranges (Siemens)
Follicle-stimulating hormone (FSH):
Follicular: 2.5–10.2 IU/L
Mid-cycle: 3.4–33.4 IU/L
Luteal: 1.5–9.1 IU/L
Post-menopausal: 23–116.3 IU/L
Luteinising hormone (LH):
Follicular: 1.9–12.5 IU/L
Mid-cycle: 8.7–76.3 IU/L
Luteal: 0.5–16.9 IU/L
Post-menopausal: 7.9–53.8 IU/L

Follicle-stimulating hormone (FSH) and luteinising hormone (LH)

Background

- Synthesis and release of the pituitary hormones FSH and LH is under the control of gonadotrophin-releasing hormone (GnRH) from the hypothalamus, and modulated by circulating gonadal steroids, e.g. oestradiol and progesterone
- FSH and LH can be used to assess the hypothalamo–pituitary–gonadal axis
- At menopause, ovarian function ceases, leading to high levels of FSH due to the removal of the negative feedback mechanisms

Indication for test

- Testing FSH and LH (ideally between day 1 and 5 of the cycle if the periods are regular):
  - fertility problems (used in conjunction with testosterone, prolactin, oestradiol and progesterone)
  - menstrual irregularities (oligo-/amenorrhoea in younger women)
  - suspected pituitary gland disorders (secondary care testing)
  - delayed puberty (secondary care testing)
- Testing only FSH (NB: testing FSH is of no value in women taking combined oral contraception or HRT, and is affected by high-dose progestogen; can be tested at any time in the cycle)
  - diagnosing premature ovarian insufficiency (POI) in women aged <40 when there are early symptoms of the menopause, including no or erratic periods
  - diagnosing menopause: only recommended in women aged 40–45 with menopausal symptoms, including a change in their menstrual cycle
    - Laboratory tests are **not** indicated in healthy women >45 who have menopause-associated symptoms
  - assessing contraceptive needs

Interpretation

Testing FSH and LH

- Causes of ↑ FSH and LH:
  - primary ovarian failure, e.g.
    - due to developmental defects: ovarian agenesis, chromosomal abnormality, e.g. Turner's syndrome
    - premature ovarian failure: radiation therapy, chemotherapy, autoimmune disease
    - chronic anovulation: PCOS, adrenal disease, thyroid disease, ovarian tumour
    - menopause
    - drugs, e.g. cimetidine, clomiphene, digitalis, levodopa
- Causes of ↓ FSH and LH:
  - secondary ovarian failure due to a pituitary or hypothalamic problem (associated with low levels of oestradiol)
  - anorexia nervosa and starvation
  - pregnancy: due to raised oestradiol levels
  - drugs, e.g. oral contraceptives, phenothiazines

- FSH and LH often need to be interpreted alongside other tests to identify the cause:

Diagnosis	Test				
	FSH	**LH**	**Oestradiol**	**Prolactin**	**Testosterone**
Hypogonadotrophic hypogonadism	↔ or ↓	↔ or ↓	↓	↔	↔
PCOS	↔	↔ or mild ↑	↔ or ↑	↔	↔ or ↑
Premature ovarian insufficiency	↑	↑	↓	↔	↔
Hyperprolactinaemia	↔ or ↓	↔ or ↓	↓	↑	↔

Adapted from BMJ Best Practice (updated 2025) *Assessment of secondary amenorrhoea.* https://bestpractice.bmj.com/topics/en-gb/1102 and Klein, D.A., Paradise, S.L. and Reeder, R.M. (2019) Amenorrhea: a systematic approach to diagnosis and management. *Am Fam Physician,* **100(1):** 39–48.

Testing only FSH

- Diagnosing premature ovarian insufficiency in women aged <40
  - diagnosis is based on raised FSH levels in the menopausal range on two blood samples taken 4–6 weeks apart (e.g. CKS NICE states FSH >30 IU/L, but this may vary with your local lab)
- Diagnosing perimenopause/menopause in women **in certain categories only**
  - **FSH testing should not be used** in otherwise healthy women (who are not using hormonal contraception) aged >45 years, with typical menopausal symptoms. Diagnose the following without laboratory testing:
    - perimenopause: if there are vasomotor symptoms and irregular periods
    - menopause: if no period for at least 12 months (and not using hormonal contraception)
    - menopause: based on symptoms in a woman without a uterus
  - **consider FSH testing** in women *not* taking combined hormonal contraception or HRT who are:
    - age >45 years with atypical symptoms
    - age 40–45 years with menopausal symptoms, including a change in menstrual cycle
    - age >50 years using progestogen-only contraception
  - single vs. repeat FSH testing guidance:
    - the Faculty of Sexual and Reproductive Healthcare (FSRH) (which became the College of Sexual and Reproductive Healthcare (CoSRH) in August 2025) states that a single elevated FSH level (>30 IU/L) indicates a degree of ovarian insufficiency, but not necessarily sterility; there is no need to repeat it
      - FSH <30 IU/L does not exclude perimenopause: levels can fluctuate greatly during the perimenopausal period

- the British Menopause Society (BMS) recommends checking for an elevated FSH level in the menopausal range on two blood samples 4–6 weeks apart
- Assessing contraceptive needs
  - CoSRH suggests restricting FSH measurement in this scenario to women age >50 years using progestogen-only contraception who are amenorrhoeic
  - women age <50 should, in general, continue contraception to age 50 years then follow the advice below
  - women age ≥50 years:
    - using combined hormonal contraception
      - stop and switch to non-hormonal methods or progestogen-only pill (POP) or implant or levonorgestrel intrauterine system, then follow the relevant advice
    - using depot medroxyprogesterone acetate (DMPA)
      - counsel regarding changing to alternative methods and follow the relevant advice
      - this may suppress FSH levels
      - FSH in the menopausal range can be confidently attributed to perimenopause/menopause; however, a result below the menopausal range cannot exclude it
      - the optimum time to measure FSH levels in a woman using DMPA is just before a repeat injection is administered
    - using progestogen-only pill or implant or levonorgestrel intrauterine system
      - if age ≥50 years with amenorrhoea and wants to stop before age 55, check FSH
        - if FSH in the menopausal range, continue contraception for 1 year and then stop (there is no need to repeat this test)
        - if FSH below the menopausal range, continue with contraception and recheck FSH after 1 year
      - stop at age 55, when natural loss of fertility can be assumed for most women

1.12.2 Oestradiol

Normal ranges (Siemens)	
Female	
Follicular:	71.6–529.2 pmol/L
Mid-cycle:	234.5–1309.1 pmol/L
Luteal:	204.8–786.1 pmol/L
Post-menopausal:	<118.2 pmol/L
(Male:	<146 pmol/L)

Background

- Oestradiol is secreted mainly by the ovary, but small amounts are produced by the adrenals and testis

Indications for test

- Testing is **unlikely to be required in primary care**
- Levels are not required for assessing menopause, as variable amounts of oestradiol are secreted in the perimenopausal period and fertile cycles may follow even with very low oestradiol levels
- NB: when managing HRT in primary care:
  - there is no recommended systemic oestradiol level in association with HRT use
  - response to treatment with HRT should be based on symptom control
  - checking serum oestradiol levels is influenced by many factors including the timing of the dose and type of assay, and cannot be assumed to be indicative of levels over a 24-hour period
  - levels can only be interpreted for people using transdermal oestradiol, not oral oestradiol
  - **routine testing of oestradiol levels is unnecessary**
- Secondary care indications for testing may include:
  - assessing ovarian status, including follicle development, for assisted reproduction protocols, e.g. *in vitro* fertilisation (IVF)
  - investigation of delayed puberty
  - HRT issues, e.g. checking for tachyphylaxis with oestrogen implants
  - investigating secondary amenorrhoea

Interpretation

Causes of ↑ oestradiol

- Ovarian tumours
- Adrenal tumours
- Precocious puberty
- Gynaecomastia

Causes of ↓ oestradiol

- Ovarian insufficiency
- Hyperprolactinaemia
- PCOS
- Anorexia nervosa
- Sheehan's syndrome

1.12.3 Progesterone

In the context of ovulation assessment, >28 nmol/L suggests ovulation has occurred (Siemens)

Background

- Progesterone is a steroid hormone mainly produced by the corpus luteum
- Levels are low during the follicular phase of the menstrual cycle

- After ovulation, progesterone production by the corpus luteum increases rapidly, reaching a maximum concentration 4–7 days after ovulation
- These levels are maintained for 4–6 days then fall to baseline levels, inducing menstruation

Indications for test

- As a marker of ovulation in the investigation of infertility
  - take blood sample 7 days before the next predicted menstruation, e.g. day 21 of a 28-day cycle
  - test may need to be repeated if the timing is incorrect
  - in women with prolonged irregular menstrual cycles, depending on the timing of menstrual periods, serum progesterone may need to be measured later, e.g. on day 28 of a 35-day cycle, and repeated weekly after that until the next menstrual cycle starts

Interpretation

- Follow the lab interpretation and comments, e.g. Siemens:
  - <16 nmol/L: ovulation unlikely to have occurred. If this is not a mid-luteal phase sample, suggest repeating approximately 7 days prior to expected menstruation
  - 16–28 nmol/L: ovulation may have occurred. If this is not a mid-luteal phase sample, suggest repeating approximately 7 days prior to expected menstruation
  - >28 nmol/L: suggests ovulation has occurred
- Refer to fertility clinic if the progesterone level is below the stated threshold for likely ovulation and the comment suggests ovulation is unlikely to have occurred

1.12.4 Testosterone

Normal ranges (Siemens)		
Testosterone	<50 years:	0.3–1.2 nmol/L
	≥50 years:	0.3–1.3 nmol/L
Sex hormone-binding globulin (SHBG)		
	<50 years:	18–138 nmol/L
	≥50 years:	24–111 nmol/L
Free androgen index (FAI)		
	20–49 years:	0.3–4.4%
	>50 years:	0.3–2.5%

Testosterone

Background

- An androgenic steroid hormone secreted from the adrenal cortex and ovaries (in females)
- In physiological concentrations, androgens have no specific effect on women
- Increased levels can lead to virilisation

- Ideally test on day 1–5 of the menstrual cycle (testosterone production increases during the early follicular phase) in the early morning (8am to 11am)

Indications for test

- Fertility investigations
- Amenorrhoea
- Hirsutism
- Virilisation
- PCOS
- Ovarian tumours
- Adrenal tumours and hyperplasia
- Hypothalamic and pituitary disorders
- Shared care monitoring of testosterone replacement in menopause

Interpretation

Causes of ↑ testosterone:

- PCOS: normal to moderately elevated; unusual for this to present >5 nmol/L
- Ovarian tumours
- Adrenal tumours and hyperplasia
- Hypothalamic and pituitary disorders

Causes of ↓ testosterone:

- Drugs, e.g. ketoconazole, metronidazole, spironolactone, cimetidine

GP management tips

- This will depend upon the presenting features and other investigations
  - refer urgently if signs of virilisation, rapidly progressing hirsutism (<1 year from onset)
- If >5 nmol/L or > twice the upper limit of normal reference range, the test should be repeated as soon as possible and if confirmed on repeat sampling; refer urgently to endocrinology

Sex hormone-binding globulin (SHBG)

Background

- 60–70% of circulating testosterone is bound to SHBG
- SHBG-bound testosterone is biologically inactive compared to its unbound 'free' form
- Note that reliable assessment of biochemical hyperandrogenism is not possible in women on hormonal contraception due to effects on SHBG and altered gonadotrophin-dependent androgen production: hormonal contraception should be stopped for at least 3 months before assessing

Indications for test

- Assessing hyperandrogenism, e.g. PCOS, hirsutism

Interpretation

- Causes of ↓ SHBG (and ↑ active testosterone):
  - PCOS: provides a surrogate measurement of the degree of hyperinsulinaemia
  - insulin resistance
  - obesity
  - hyperprolactinaemia
  - hypothyroidism
- Causes of ↑ SHBG (and ↓ active testosterone):
  - oestrogen
  - pregnancy
  - hyperthyroidism
  - excess alcohol
  - liver disease
  - anticonvulsants

Free androgen index (FAI)

Background

- Free androgen index (FAI) = $\dfrac{\text{total testosterone (nmol/L)} \times 100}{\text{SHBG (nmol/L)}}$
- This is a simple method of estimating the circulating free testosterone
- It may be unreliable in situations where there are extreme abnormalities in SHBG, or albumin is not in range
- Note that reliable assessment of biochemical hyperandrogenism is not possible in women on hormonal contraception due to effects on SHBG and altered gonadotrophin-dependent androgen production: hormonal contraception should be stopped for at least 3 months before assessing

Indications for test

- Assessing hyperandrogenism

Interpretation

- FAI is more sensitive at detecting hyperandrogenism than total testosterone and may be helpful in assessing androgen status where total testosterone is in the upper half of the reference range
  - if total testosterone is in the lower part of the reference range, FAI is generally not ↑
- Normal or elevated in women with PCOS (≥5)
  - as PCOS is associated with ↓ SHBG, this increases the FAI (i.e. free active hormone), while total testosterone can remain normal

1.12.5 Cancer antigen 125 (CA125)

Normal range <36 kU/L (Siemens)

Background

- Used to investigate possible symptoms of ovarian cancer
- Refer as urgent suspected cancer (gynaecology) if there is ascites or a pelvic or abdominal mass (not caused by known fibroids)

Indication for test

If the examination is normal (i.e. no ascites, pelvic/abdominal mass):
- Test CA125 in any woman (particularly if age >50 years) if any of the following symptoms are persistent or frequent (particularly >12 times per month):
  - abdominal distension (bloating)
  - feeling full (early satiety) and/or loss of appetite
  - pelvic or abdominal pain
  - increased urinary urgency and/or frequency
  - in any woman age >50 years if she has had symptoms suggestive of IBS within the last 12 months (IBS rarely presents for the first time in women of this age)
- Consider testing CA125 in any woman who reports:
  - any unexplained weight loss, malaise/fatigue or change in bowel habit
  - abnormal or postmenopausal bleeding
  - GI symptoms, such as dyspepsia, nausea or bowel obstruction
  - shortness of breath, e.g. due to pleural effusion

Interpretation

- CA125 ≥36 kU/L
  - arrange an urgent abdomen and pelvis ultrasound scan
    - if the ultrasound is suggestive of ovarian cancer, refer as urgent suspected cancer (gynaecology)
- CA125 <36 kU/L, or CA125 ≥36 kU/L but with a normal ultrasound:
  - consider other causes:
    - conditions with similar symptoms
      - other cancers, e.g. cervix, uterus, rectum and bladder
      - abdominal distension/bloating: fibroids, ascites, adenomyosis
      - early satiety: gastric cancer
      - urinary frequency/urgency: recurrent UTIs
      - altered bowel habit: IBS, constipation, coeliac disease, IBD, GI infection
      - abdominal pain/discomfort: adhesions, pelvic inflammatory disease (PID), diverticular disease, chronic pancreatitis, gallstones
    - other causes of ↑ CA125
      - peritoneal trauma, disease or irritation
      - other cancers, e.g. primary peritoneal, lung and pancreatic cancer
      - endometriosis

- PID
  - ovarian cyst torsion, rupture or haemorrhage
  - pregnancy
  - heart failure
- o if no other clinical cause is apparent, advise patient to return for review if the symptoms become more frequent and/or persistent

1.12.6 Human chorionic gonadotrophin (hCG)

Blood normal range: <10 IU/L (Siemens)

Background

- hCG is secreted by the placenta in pregnancy, and thus forms the basis for urine pregnancy testing: **point-of-care urine tests should suffice in primary care**
- For patients under the care of the Early Pregnancy Unit, serum hCG may be used to monitor progression of a pregnancy (not usually tested in primary care)
- hCG can be used as a tumour marker when germ cell tumours are suspected, and can be present in non-germ cell tumours, e.g. small cell carcinoma of the lung (not tested in primary care)

Indications for test

- To confirm or exclude pregnancy
  - o for practical purposes, this is generally done via point-of-care urine tests
    - ■ hormone levels are highest first thing in the morning, so a first-pass morning urine sample is best; however, this can be a random sample

Interpretation

- Blood hCG used as a pregnancy test
  - o >25 IU/L would normally indicate a positive pregnancy test
  - o NB: a result of <25 IU/L does not exclude early pregnancy
- Urine hCG
  - o a routine pregnancy test has a sensitivity of 25 IU/L

Causes of false positive results

- Blood or protein in the urine
- Drugs, e.g. anticonvulsant, anti-Parkinson drugs, hypnotics and tranquillisers

Causes of false negative results

- Tests performed too early in pregnancy: it takes 7–10 days after conception for the test to become positive
- Drugs, e.g. diuretics and promethazine
- Very dilute urine (drinking large volumes of fluid before the sample should be avoided)

GP management tips

- Interval hCG blood testing should be performed in secondary care in cases of pregnancy of unknown location or in those who have symptoms such as bleeding in early pregnancy, as checking hCG is typically paired with ultrasound evaluation
- In the first 8 weeks, blood hCG normally doubles every 2 days
- Those who have hCG levels that plateau prior to 8 weeks or that fail to double commonly have a non-viable pregnancy (intra-uterine or extra-uterine)
- hCG will drop rapidly following a miscarriage: if hCG does not fall to undetectable levels, it may indicate remaining hCG-producing tissue that will need to be removed
- Following miscarriage it may take 3–4 weeks for hCG to return to non-pregnant levels
- In all non-pregnant patients, other malignancies should be evaluated as a source of persistently positive hCG testing by secondary care

References

References to support all aspects of testing and management guidance can be found, broken up by section, by scanning the QR code below or clicking on the Resources tab on the page for this book at www.scionpublishing.com/lab_results

Chapter 2

Haematology

ABNORMAL RESULTS

Follow your local reference ranges, clinical pathways, management and referral guidance. This guidance is not a substitute for individual clinical judgement. Reference ranges will vary according to the assay used by laboratories. Those provided are examples and may vary in your locality.

2.1 Full blood count

2.1.1 Haemoglobin

Low haemoglobin (anaemia) (♂ Hb <130 g/L; ♀ Hb <115 g/L)

Normal range: ♂ 130–180 g/L; ♀ 115–165 g/L   MCV: 80–100 fL

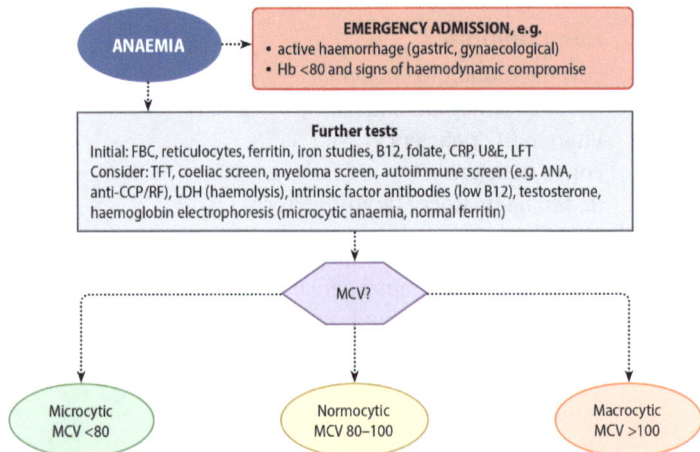

Microcytic anaemia (MCV <80 fL)

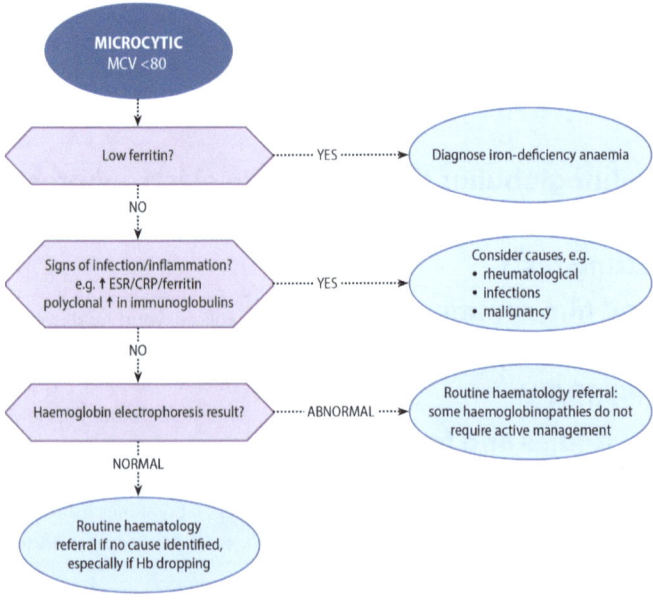

Normocytic anaemia (MCV 80–100 fL)

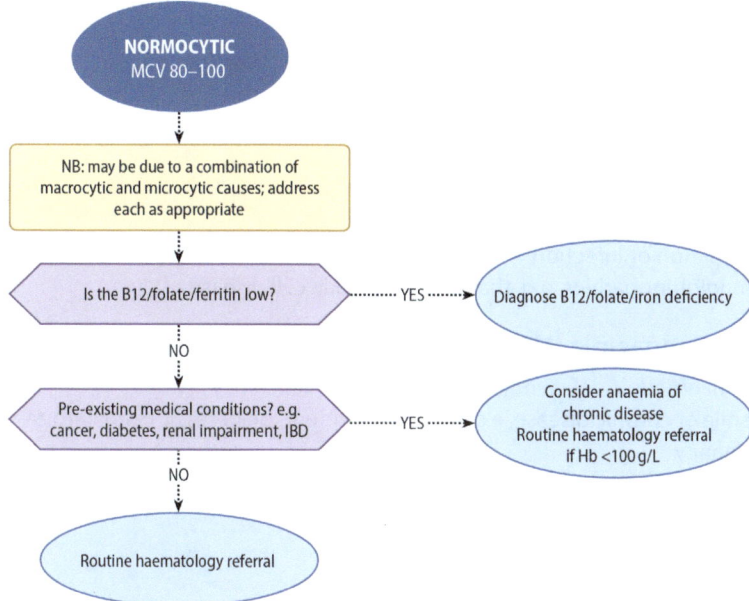

Macrocytic anaemia (MCV >100 fL)

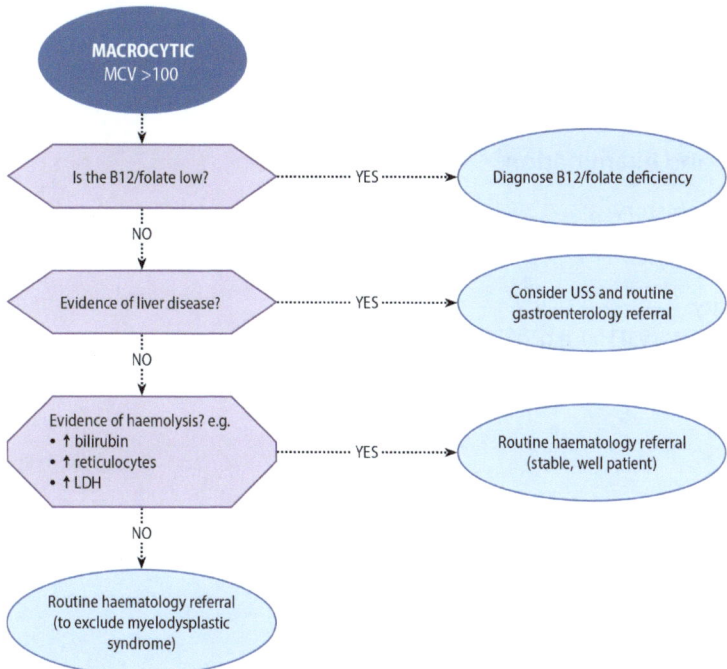

Background

- Anaemia can be multifactorial: note a combination of causes may result in a mixed picture
- The MCV is a useful starting point to guide further investigation

Causes

Microcytic anaemia (MCV <80 fL)

- Iron-deficiency anaemia (IDA)
- Inflammation or infection
- Haemoglobinopathies, e.g. thalassaemia, sickle cell disease

Normocytic anaemia (MCV 80–100 fL)

- Mixed haematinic deficiency, e.g. iron and B12 deficiency
- Anaemia of chronic disease, e.g. renal impairment, diabetes, ↓ testosterone
- Malignancy
- Acute blood loss

Macrocytic anaemia (MCV >100 fL)

- ↓ B12
- ↓ folate
- Alcohol excess
- Liver disease
- Hypothyroidism
- Medication, e.g. hydroxycarbamide, methotrexate
- Pregnancy
- Haemolysis
- Bone marrow disorder, e.g. myelodysplasia

History and examination

- Bleeding history
- Chronic disease history, e.g. renal failure, liver disease, inflammatory bowel disease (IBD)
- Ethnicity
- Family history (FHx), e.g. of bleeding disorder

- Lifestyle review, e.g. diet, alcohol
- Medication, e.g. non-steroidal anti-inflammatory drugs (NSAIDs), steroids
- Significant past medical history e.g. gastritis, fibroids
- Symptoms and signs of anaemia, e.g. shortness of breath, fatigue, dizziness, pallor, jaundice, koilonychia, angular cheilosis, glossitis, alopecia
- Symptoms and signs of recurrent infections, ulcers, recent viral illness, autoimmune or connective tissue disorders
- Symptoms and signs of malignancy, e.g. bowel symptoms, post-menopausal bleeding, haemoptysis, lymphadenopathy and hepatosplenomegaly, 'B symptoms' (fever, drenching night sweats, weight loss >10% in previous 6 months), weight loss

Investigations

- Initial:
  - full blood count (FBC) repeat
  - reticulocytes
  - ferritin, iron studies
  - B12, folate
  - CRP
  - U&E, liver function test (LFT)
- Consider:
  - thyroid function test (TFT)
  - coeliac screen
  - myeloma screen
  - lactate dehydrogenase (LDH) (haemolysis)
  - intrinsic factor antibodies (low B12, if not had previously and no known GI surgery that could cause malabsorption)
  - autoimmune screen, e.g. ANA, anti-CCP/RF (as per local guidance)
  - testosterone
  - haemoglobin electrophoresis (if microcytic anaemia, normal ferritin levels and not previously checked)
  - urine dip (for blood)
  - stool parasites (if relevant travel history and/or eosinophilia)
  - faecal immunochemical test (FIT): offer to all with IDA, or age ≥60 and non-IDA
  - liver ultrasound scan (USS) (liver disease)
  - pelvis USS: women age ≥55 with anaemia and visible haematuria (endometrial cancer)
  - routine oesophagogastroduodenoscopy (OGD): age ≥55 with anaemia and upper abdominal pain (oesophageal or stomach cancer)

Referral

Emergency admission

- Acutely unwell, e.g. active haemorrhage, Hb <80 and haemodynamic compromise
- ↓ B12/folate with neurological symptoms (hypokalaemia can develop during initial replacement of severe B12 deficiency)
- Unexplained progressive symptomatic anaemia
- Sickle cell crisis, e.g. severe pain, acute chest syndrome, stroke, priapism

Urgent suspected cancer

- Suspected malignancy (relevant specialty)
- Suspected haematological malignancy (haematology), e.g.
  - abnormal blood film, e.g. leucoerythroblastic picture (presence of immature white cells and nucleated red blood cells)
  - anaemia with accompanying cytopenia but normal B12, folate and ferritin
  - associated hepatosplenomegaly, lymphadenopathy

Routine outpatient

- Persistent unexplained anaemia with Hb ≤100 g/L (haematology)
- Unresponsive to or unable to tolerate corrective therapy (relevant specialty)
- Anaemia of chronic disease (relevant specialty as needed)
- Renal anaemia (nephrology)
- Persistent unexplained MCV >105 (haematology)
- Interpreting haemoglobin electrophoresis results; not all haemoglobinopathies need active management, e.g. beta thalassaemia trait, sickle cell trait and alpha thalassaemia trait (haematology)
- Suspected haemolysis (haematology)

Advice & Guidance

- Diagnostic uncertainty (relevant specialty)

GP management tips

- Consider interval monitoring of patients who are elderly/frail with a mild, unexplained, asymptomatic anaemia (Hb >100 g/L) following exclusion of reversible causes
- Uncomplicated B12 or folate deficiency does not require referral
- IDA is generally not managed by haematology
- Haemoglobinopathy screening: document testing result clearly (no need for repeat testing)

Iron-deficiency anaemia (IDA)

Background

- Defined as ↓ red blood cell production due to ↓ body iron stores
- Blood findings: ↓ haemoglobin, ↓ MCV, serum ferritin level <30 µg/L, ↓ transferrin saturation
- Blood film: microcytic, hypochromic red cells, pencil cells and thrombocytosis
- Interpreting ferritin levels
  - ferritin is the most specific test for iron deficiency in the absence of inflammation
  - the lower limit of normal for most labs is between 15 and 30 µg/L
    - ferritin <15 µg/L is indicative of absent iron stores (specificity 0.99)
    - ferritin <30 µg/L is indicative of low body iron stores
  - ferritin is an acute phase protein, so apparently normal levels may occur with iron deficiency in the context of an inflammatory disease process
  - a cut-off of 45 µg/L has been suggested as providing the optimal trade-off between sensitivity and specificity for iron deficiency in practice (specificity of 0.92); figures below this may warrant consideration of GI investigation, especially in the context of a chronic inflammatory process with anaemia
  - a value >150 µg/L is unlikely to occur with absolute iron deficiency, even in the presence of inflammation

Causes

- Blood loss, e.g. gastrointestinal, gynaecological or urological, blood donor
- Poor dietary iron intake, e.g. vegetarian
- Malabsorption, e.g. coeliac, gastrectomy
- Increased requirements, e.g. myeloproliferative neoplasms
- Pregnancy
- Medication, e.g. aspirin, NSAIDs, selective serotonin reuptake inhibitors (SSRIs), clopidogrel, corticosteroids, long-term PPI

Investigations

- Initial tests
  - FBC, ferritin, iron studies, B12, folate, coeliac screen, ESR/CRP, reticulocytes
  - FIT
  - urine dip (for blood)
- Consider:
  - stool parasite (if relevant travel history and/or eosinophilia)

Referral

IDA is generally not managed by haematology

Emergency admission

- Acutely unwell, e.g. active haemorrhage, Hb <80 and haemodynamic compromise
- Unexplained progressive symptomatic anaemia

Urgent suspected cancer

- Suspected malignancy (relevant specialty)
  - FIT result of ≥10 µg Hb/g faeces (colorectal)
  - post-menopausal bleeding in women age ≥55 (gynaecology; endometrial cancer)
  - post-menopausal bleeding in women age <55 (consider gynaecology referral; endometrial cancer)

Urgent outpatient (gastroenterology)

NB: check local referral protocols if meets urgent suspected cancer pathway criteria
- Men and post-menopausal women with newly diagnosed IDA unless they have overt non-GI bleeding
  - men with Hb <120 g/L and post-menopausal women with Hb <100 g/L should be investigated more urgently, as lower levels of Hb suggest more serious disease (consider urgent suspected cancer referral)
- All people age ≥50 with marked anaemia, or a significant FHx of colorectal carcinoma, even if coeliac disease is found
- Premenopausal women if they are age <50 and have colonic symptoms, a strong FHx (two affected 1st-degree relatives or just one 1st-degree relative affected before the age of 50) of GI cancer, persistent IDA despite treatment, or if they do not menstruate, e.g. hysterectomy

Routine outpatient

- Unable to tolerate corrective therapy, for possible IV iron therapy (gastroenterology)
- Unresponsive to initial therapy, i.e. Hb increase <20 g/L after 4 weeks, or develops anaemia again without an obvious underlying cause (gastroenterology)
- Positive coeliac screen (gastroenterology)
- Menorrhagia unresponsive to medical management (gynaecology)

GP management tips

- Do not wait for investigations to be carried out before prescribing iron supplements, e.g. one tablet daily of oral ferrous sulfate / fumarate / gluconate, unless colonoscopy imminent
- If not tolerated, reduce the dose to one tablet on alternate days, or consider alternative oral preparations, e.g. oral ferric maltol
- Monitor to ensure adequate response to treatment:
  - recheck FBC in the first 4 weeks of treatment: Hb should rise by about 20 g/L
  - if there is a response, check FBC at 2–4 months to ensure Hb has normalised
  - continue iron treatment for a further 3 months to replenish stores, then stop
  - monitor FBC periodically, e.g. every 6 months
  - if Hb drops below normal, prescribe iron supplements
- Further investigation is only necessary if Hb cannot be maintained this way or if there is any evidence of an active undiagnosed pathology, e.g.
  - ongoing weight loss
  - chronic unexplained diarrhoea

- o persistently ↑ inflammatory markers
- o persistence or recurrence of IDA
- Consider ongoing prophylactic iron (e.g. 200 mg ferrous sulfate daily), monitoring FBC every 6–12 months, in those at particular risk of IDA, e.g.
  - o recurring anaemia in elderly and further tests are not indicated or appropriate
  - o plant-based diets
  - o malabsorption, e.g. coeliac disease, gastrectomy
  - o menorrhagia
- Iron turns the stool black, so melaena may be difficult to report once iron treatment is started
- Advise food sources rich in iron:
  - o red meats (beef, lamb and pork) and offal
  - o fish and poultry
  - o plant-based sources: pulses and legumes (e.g. beans, peas and lentils), dark green vegetables (e.g. spinach, kale and broccoli), nuts and seeds
  - o some foods are fortified with iron, e.g. all UK-sold bread (except wholemeal) must be fortified; many breakfast cereals are also fortified
  - o absorption is enhanced with animal protein foods and vitamin C, but reduced by bran-containing cereals and tannins in tea and coffee
- Iron deficiency without anaemia
  - o before iron-deficiency anaemia develops, there is an initial phase where body iron stores are depleted, resulting in low ferritin levels with a normal Hb concentration
  - o the prevalence of significant underlying GI pathology, especially malignancy, is low
  - o thus, in the absence of other pointers, GI investigation generally is not warranted in premenopausal women; the cause is likely to be menstrual blood loss and/or recent pregnancy
  - o the threshold for investigation of iron deficiency without anaemia should be low in men, postmenopausal women, and those with GI symptoms or a FHx of GI pathology

Vitamin B12 deficiency (<180 ng/L: confirmed deficiency)

Background

- Blood findings: macrocytic anaemia with megaloblastic changes (hyper-segmented neutrophils on blood film)
- There is no gold standard test for measuring vitamin B12 deficiency, but the likelihood of deficiency can be determined by measuring serum cobalamin (total B12)
  - o a serum cobalamin of <200 ng/L is sensitive enough to diagnose 97% with vitamin B12 deficiency
- NICE recommends these thresholds to interpret test results (serum cobalamin):
  - o <180 ng/L   confirmed deficiency
  - o 180–350 ng/L   possible deficiency
  - o >350 ng/L   unlikely deficiency

Causes

- Poor absorption, e.g. pernicious anaemia, gastrectomy, IBD
- Medication, e.g. PPI, H_2 receptor antagonists, colchicine, metformin, oral contraceptive pill (OCP), recreational nitrous oxide use
- Dietary, e.g. malnutrition, vegan diet

Investigations

- Initial tests
  - o FBC, B12, folate, coeliac screen
  - o intrinsic factor antibodies (if not had previously and no known GI surgery that could cause malabsorption)
- Consider:
  - o LFT, TFT (non-megaloblastic causes of macrocytosis)
  - o ferritin, iron studies (exclude concurrent deficiency)

Referral

Uncomplicated B12 deficiency does not require referral to haematology

Emergency admission

- ↓ B12 with neurological symptoms (treatment can cause hypokalaemia so requires regular monitoring)

Urgent suspected cancer

- Known pernicious anaemia and a suspicion of gastric cancer (gastroenterology)
- Suspected blood malignancy (haematology)

Routine outpatient

- Suspected malabsorption, IBD, positive coeliac screen (gastroenterology)
- Nutritional advice (dietitian)
- Cause of deficiency unclear after investigations, not responding to treatment, MCV >105 (haematology)

Advice & Guidance

- Recreational nitrous oxide use requires different tests: serum methylmalonic acid (MMA) can be used as the initial test, or plasma homocysteine (secondary care tests)

GP management tips

- Medication-induced or nitrous oxide-related B12 deficiency:
  - o offer either intramuscular (IM) or oral B12 replacement while using medication
  - o review if the medication can be stopped; encourage stopping nitrous oxide use
  - o review B12 replacement if stopped and deficiency symptoms have resolved
- Suspected dietary cause:
  - o review dietary B12 intake and consider oral B12 replacement. B12 sources:

- meat, egg and dairy products
  - B12-fortified plant foods: yeast extract, fortified plant-based drinks and alternatives to yogurt and most fortified breakfast cereals
  - o review OTC vitamin use
    - oral supplement should contain at least one of the following: cyanocobalamin, methylcobalamin or adenosylcobalamin
  - o review concurrent causes of possible B12 deficiency
  - o consider IM B12 injections instead of oral if:
    - concurrent condition which may affect quality of life, e.g. ataxia or anaemia
    - concerns about oral treatment concordance, e.g. frailty, cognitive impairment
- Cause unknown:
  - o offer B12 replacement, considering oral versus IM replacement and review response
- If hydroxocobalamin injection is necessary, initially administer 1 mg IM three times a week for 2 weeks
- The maintenance dose depends on whether the deficiency is diet-related or not
  - o if not thought to be diet-related:
    - give hydroxocobalamin 1 mg IM every 2–3 months for life
    - alternatively, consider daily large oral doses (500–1000 µg)
  - o if thought to be diet-related
    - oral cyanocobalamin tablets 50–150 µg OD between meals
    - alternatively twice-yearly hydroxocobalamin 1 mg IM
    - in vegans, treatment may need to be lifelong, whereas in other people with dietary deficiency replacement, treatment can be stopped once the B12 levels have corrected and diet has improved
- Monitoring response; check FBC and reticulocytes:
  - o within 7–10 days of starting treatment
    - a ↑ in Hb and ↑ in reticulocyte count above the normal range indicates treatment is working
  - o after 8 weeks of treatment (FBC, reticulocytes)
    - blood counts and MCV should have normalised
    - measure ferritin/iron studies and folate to ensure other deficiencies not masked
- Measuring cobalamin levels is unhelpful as levels increase with treatment regardless of how effective it is, and retesting is not usually required; however, cobalamin can be:
  - o measured 1–2 months after starting treatment if there is no response
  - o rechecked if a lack of treatment compliance is suspected, anaemia recurs, or neurological symptoms do not improve or progress
- Neurological recovery may take time: improvement begins within 1 week and complete resolution usually occurs between 6 and 12 weeks

Folate deficiency (<3 μg/L)

Background

- Blood findings: macrocytic anaemia, megaloblastic changes (hyper-segmented neutrophils)
- There is no clear consensus on the level of serum folate that indicates deficiency. Conventionally, a serum folate <3 μg/L is used as a guideline, as the risk of megaloblastic anaemia greatly increases below this level

Causes

- Malabsorption, e.g. coeliac disease, surgery, IBD
- Dietary, e.g. malnutrition, vegan diet, excess alcohol
- Medication, e.g. nitrofurantoin, trimethoprim, anticonvulsants, sulfasalazine, methotrexate
- Increased requirements
  - pregnancy
  - malignancy
  - blood disorders, e.g. haemolytic anaemia, sickle cell anaemia
  - inflammatory diseases, e.g. TB
  - exfoliative skin diseases
- Excessive urinary excretion, e.g. heart failure, liver disease, renal disease

Investigations

- Initial tests
  - FBC, B12, folate, coeliac screen
- Consider:
  - LFT, TFT (non-megaloblastic causes of macrocytosis)
  - ferritin, iron studies (exclude concurrent deficiency)

Referral

Uncomplicated folate deficiency does not require referral to haematology

Emergency admission

- ↓ folate with neurological symptoms

Urgent suspected cancer

- Suspected blood malignancy (haematology)

Routine outpatient

- Suspected malabsorption, IBD, positive coeliac screen (gastroenterology)
- Nutritional advice (dietitian)
- Cause of deficiency unclear after investigations, not responding to treatment, MCV >105 (haematology)

GP management tips

- Ensure B12 levels are normal or replaced **before** treating to avoid development of sub-acute combined degeneration of the cord
- Dietary sources: asparagus, broccoli, brown rice, brussels sprouts, chickpeas, peas
- Prescribe oral folic acid 5 mg daily for 4 months; may be required for longer (even for life) if the underlying cause of deficiency is persistent
- Monitoring response; check FBC and reticulocytes:
  - within 7–10 days of starting treatment
    - a ↑ in Hb and ↑ in reticulocyte count above the normal range indicates treatment is working
  - after 8 weeks of treatment (FBC, reticulocytes)
    - blood counts and MCV should have normalised
  - on completion of folic acid treatment to confirm response

Raised haematocrit (erythrocytosis)

Normal ranges: ♂ 0.40–0.52 L/L (40–52%); ♀ 0.37–0.48 L/L (37–48%)

Background

- Raised haematocrit can be due to ↑ haemoglobin (true erythrocytosis) or ↓ plasma volume (apparent erythrocytosis)
- The term 'polycythaemia' should be reserved for overproduction of red cells due to a bone marrow problem, e.g. polycythaemia rubra vera

Causes

- Primary erythrocytosis
  - polycythaemia rubra vera (97% have *JAK2* gene mutation)
- Secondary erythrocytosis
  - congenital (rare)
  - acquired
    - hypoxia from respiratory or cardiac disease
    - medication, e.g. testosterone, anabolic steroids
    - lifestyle, e.g. obesity, alcohol excess, smoking, hypertension
  - abnormal erythropoietin production
    - renal issues
    - tumour, e.g. fibroids, hepatocellular and renal cell carcinoma
- Apparent erythrocytosis
  - dehydration
  - medication, e.g. diuretics

History and examination

- Aquagenic pruritus (itching after getting body wet)

- Symptoms of hyperviscosity, e.g. headaches, visual disturbances, neurological symptoms, weakness
- Examination: oxygen saturations, blood pressure, BMI

Investigations

- Initial:
  - full blood count (FBC) (uncuffed sample, minimum interval 1 week, non-fasted)
  - blood film
  - U&E, LFT, bone profile
  - HbA1c
  - ferritin/iron studies (iron deficiency can mask the degree of erythrocytosis)
  - urine dip (exclude renal issues, e.g. proteinuria, haematuria)
- Consider:
  - chest X-ray (CXR), spirometry (suspected respiratory cause)
  - USS abdomen

Referral

Emergency admission

- ↑haematocrit (♂ >0.52, ♀ >0.48) and symptoms of hyperviscosity

Urgent outpatient

- New extreme ↑haematocrit (♂ >0.60, ♀ >0.56) in the absence of congenital cyanotic heart disease (haematology)
- ↑haematocrit (♂ >0.52, ♀ >0.48) in association with recent (last 3 months) arterial or venous thrombosis (including DVT/PE, CVA/TIA, MI/unstable angina, PVD) (haematology)

Routine outpatient

- Persistent unexplained ↑haematocrit (♂ >0.52, ♀ >0.48) (two tests >6 weeks apart) (haematology)
- ↑haematocrit, but ↓MCV or ferritin: could be iron-deficient polycythaemia vera; do not give iron therapy in this situation as it will worsen the erythrocytosis (haematology)
- Suspected hypoxic respiratory disease (respiratory)
- Suspected heart failure (cardiology)

GP management tips

- Cardiovascular risk factors (including hyperlipidaemia, smoking, hypertension and diabetes) should be managed in all with erythrocytosis of any cause

2.1.2 White cell count

The white cell count measures the total number of white blood cells per volume of blood. The differential white cell count examines the sub-types of white blood cells present: neutrophils, lymphocytes, basophils, eosinophils and monocytes.

Low neutrophils (neutropenia) (neutrophils $<1.5 \times 10^9$/L)

Normal range: 1.5–8.0×10^9/L

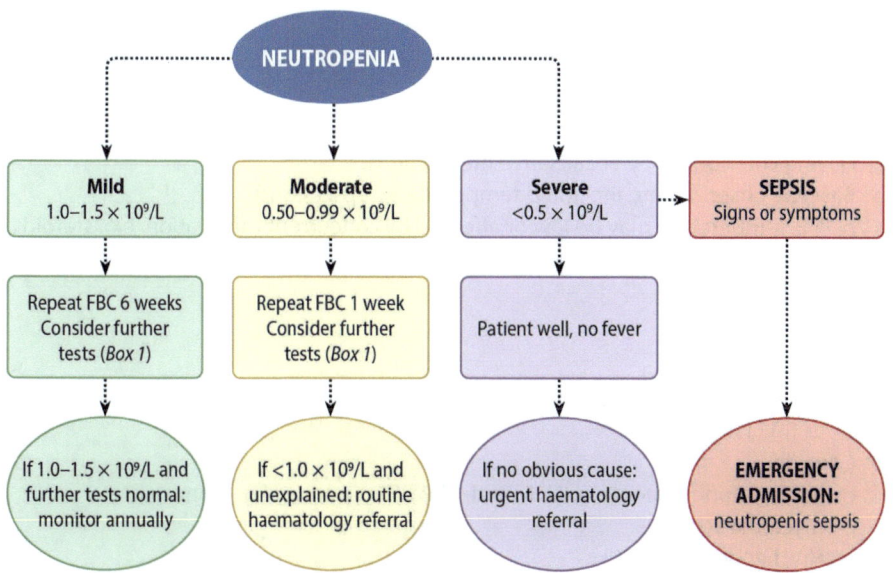

NEUTROPENIA

| **Mild** 1.0–1.5×10^9/L | **Moderate** 0.50–0.99×10^9/L | **Severe** $<0.5 \times 10^9$/L | **SEPSIS** Signs or symptoms |

Repeat FBC 6 weeks Consider further tests (*Box 1*)

Repeat FBC 1 week Consider further tests (*Box 1*)

Patient well, no fever

If 1.0–1.5×10^9/L and further tests normal: monitor annually

If $<1.0 \times 10^9$/L and unexplained: routine haematology referral

If no obvious cause: urgent haematology referral

EMERGENCY ADMISSION: neutropenic sepsis

Box 1 Further tests
Initial: Blood film, LFT, TFT, B12, folate
Consider: Autoimmune screen (e.g. ANA, anti-CCP/RF), myeloma screen, HIV, hepatitis B & C

Background

- Neutropenia secondary to chemotherapy should be referred for acute oncology review: neutropenic sepsis is a medical emergency
- There is ↑ risk of more serious infection when $<1.0 \times 10^9$/L, and especially when $<0.5 \times 10^9$/L

Causes

- Medication, e.g. carbimazole, clozapine, clotrimazole, chemotherapy, phenytoin
- Viral infections, e.g. Epstein–Barr virus (EBV), hepatitis B and C, HIV (may take weeks to resolve)
- Sepsis

- Autoimmune disease, e.g. rheumatoid arthritis (RA), systemic lupus erythematosus (SLE)
- $\downarrow$ B12 or $\downarrow$ folate
- Ethnic variations, e.g. people of African or Middle Eastern descent frequently have a constitutional neutropenia, usually $>1.0 \times 10^9$/L, that is of no clinical consequence. This is a diagnosis of exclusion after ruling out other causes and seeing a persistent $\downarrow$ count without increased risk of infection
- Hypersplenism
- Thyroid dysfunction
- Nutritional deficiencies, e.g. anorexia nervosa
- Bone marrow issues, e.g. myelodysplasia, aplastic anaemia, acute leukaemia, myeloma

History and examination

- Having chemotherapy or causative medications?
- Baseline observations, including temperature (sepsis signs)
  - NB: temperature may be low or affected by concurrent medication, e.g. steroids

Investigations

- Initial:
  - blood film
  - B12, folate
  - LFT, TFT
- Consider:
  - autoimmune screen, e.g. ANA, anti-CCP/RF (as per local guidance)
  - myeloma screen
  - HIV, hepatitis B and C

Referral

Emergency admission

- Neutrophil $<0.5 \times 10^9$/L and sepsis
- Unwell patient with **any** severity of neutropenia

Urgent suspected cancer

- Suspected blood malignancy, e.g. associated cytopenia, hepatosplenomegaly, lymphadenopathy (haematology)

Urgent outpatient

- Neutrophil $<0.5 \times 10^9$/L, but systemically well (significant risk of infection) (haematology)

Routine outpatient

- Persistently unexplained neutropenia $<1.0 \times 10^9$/L (two tests >6 weeks apart) (haematology)

Low lymphocytes (lymphopenia) (lymphocyte count <1.5 × 10⁹/L)

Normal range: 1.5–5.0 × 10⁹/L

Background

- Grading of severity:
  - mild: 1.0–1.5 × 10⁹/L
  - moderate: 0.50–0.99 × 10⁹/L
  - severe: <0.5 × 10⁹/L
- Lymphopenia is a common, non-specific and often transient finding which increases in frequency with older age and comorbidities
- It is more often of no pathological significance: however, HIV infection is commonly associated with lymphopenia
- Rarely associated with haematological conditions, but can be observed in lymphoproliferative disorders

Causes

- Increasing age
- Infection, e.g. acute or chronic (HIV, hepatitis B and C, TB)
- Medication, e.g. steroids, immunosuppressants, chemotherapy, methotrexate, azathioprine
- Systemic disorders, e.g. autoimmune disease, IBD, sarcoidosis
- Malignancy, e.g. lymphoproliferative disorders, solid organ malignancies
- Stress, e.g. exercise, malnutrition, alcohol, surgery, radiotherapy
- Chronic disease, e.g. cardiac failure, renal failure
- Primary immunodeficiency

History and examination

- Examine for lymphadenopathy and hepatosplenomegaly
- Ask about B symptoms
- Symptoms and signs of recurrent infections, ulcers, recent viral illness, autoimmune or connective tissue disorders

Investigations

- Initial:
  - blood film
  - B12, folate
  - U&E, LFT
- Consider:
  - myeloma screen
  - autoimmune screen, e.g. ANA, anti-CCP/RF (as per local guidance)
  - HIV, hepatitis B and C

Referral

Urgent suspected cancer

- Suspected malignancy (relevant specialty)

Urgent outpatient

- Severe lymphopenia (<0.5 × 10^9/L), as may predispose to opportunistic infections, e.g. *Pneumocystis* pneumonia, oesophageal candidiasis, herpes zoster (haematology)

Routine outpatient

- Diagnostic uncertainty with persistent moderate lymphopenia >6 months (haematology)
- Lymphopenia with recurrent infections and HIV negative, consider immunodeficiency issue and checking immunoglobulins (immunology)
- Suspected autoimmune disease (rheumatology)

GP management tips

- Mild lymphopenia (1.0–1.5 × 10^9/L), well patient: no further action
- Well patient, age >70 and lymphocytes >0.5 × 10^9/L: no further action
- Moderate lymphopenia (0.50–0.99 × 10^9/L), well patient:
  - consider further investigations
  - if no cause identified, repeat FBC at 6 months
    - if no change in count and patient remains well, no need to investigate further
    - consider routine haematology referral if there are any changes/concerns

High white cell count (leucocytosis) (white cell count >11 × 10^9/L)

Normal range: 3.6–11.0 × 10^9/L

Background

- The differential is wide-ranging, from a normal reaction to infection to haematological malignancies

Causes

- Infection (especially bacterial)
- Inflammation
- Stress events, e.g. trauma, MI
- Malignancy, e.g. haematological or solid tumour
- Autoimmune disease
- Smoking (minor non-specific leucocytosis or neutrophilia is often seen)

History and examination

- Examine for lymphadenopathy and hepatosplenomegaly
- Ask about B symptoms
- Symptoms and signs of infection, autoimmune or connective tissue disorders

Investigations

- Initial:
  - assess white cell count (WCC) differential (if lymphocytosis and neutrophilia present, reactive cause is more likely)
  - blood film
  - ESR/CRP
- Consider:
  - autoimmune screen, e.g. ANA, anti-CCP/RF (as per local guidance)
  - HIV, hepatitis B and C

Referral

Emergency admission

- New suspected acute leukaemia (likely to be contacted by lab about the result)
- New suspected chronic myeloid leukaemia (CML) with WCC >100 × 10⁹/L or hyperviscosity symptoms (likely to be contacted by lab about the result)
- Acutely unwell patient, e.g. with severe infection / sepsis

Urgent suspected cancer

- New CML without emergency admission criteria (haematology)
- Age ≥60 and ↑ WCC with unexplained non-visible haematuria (bladder cancer, urology)
- Suspected malignancy (relevant specialty)

Urgent outpatient

- Unexplained leucocytosis with WCC >50 × 10⁹/L (haematology)

Routine outpatient

- Unexplained persistent raised levels (two tests >6 weeks apart) (haematology)
  - WCC: >20 × 10⁹/L
  - neutrophilia: >15 × 10⁹/L
  - lymphocytes: >5 × 10⁹/L
  - eosinophilia: >1.5 × 10⁹/L
  - monocytosis: >1 × 10⁹/L
  - basophilia: >0.2 × 10⁹/L

High neutrophils (neutrophilia) (neutrophils >8 × 10⁹/L)

Normal range: 1.5–8.0 × 10⁹/L

Background

- Usually a reactive phenomenon
- It is unusual for a reactive neutrophilia to be above 100×10^9/L

Causes

- Infection (especially bacterial)
- Inflammation
- Stress events, e.g. trauma, myocardial infarction (MI)
- Medication, e.g. steroids, lithium
- Pregnancy
- Smoking (minor non-specific leucocytosis or neutrophilia is often seen)
- Hyposplenism
- Autoimmune disease
- Malignancy, e.g. haematological or solid tumour

History and examination

- Examine for lymphadenopathy and hepatosplenomegaly
- Ask about B symptoms
- Symptoms and signs of infection, autoimmune or connective tissue disorders
- Travel history

Investigations

- Initial:
  - blood film
  - CRP/ESR
  - U&E, LFT
- Consider:
  - autoimmune screen, e.g. ANA, anti-CCP/RF (as per local guidance)
  - prostate-specific antigen (PSA)

Referral

Emergency admission

- Acutely unwell patient, e.g. with severe infection/sepsis
- New suspected CML with WCC >100×10^9/L or hyperviscosity symptoms (likely to be contacted by lab about the result)

Urgent suspected cancer

- Suspected haematological malignancy, e.g. abnormal blood film, splenomegaly (haematology)
- Suspected malignancy (relevant specialty)

Urgent outpatient

- Unexplained inflammatory process (relevant specialty)

Routine outpatient

- Unexplained persistent neutrophilia >15 × 10⁹/L (two tests >6 weeks apart) (haematology)

High lymphocytes (lymphocytosis) (lymphocytes >5 × 10⁹/L)

Normal range: 1.5–5.0 × 10⁹/L

Background

- Usually a reactive phenomenon, but it is important to check a blood film

Causes

- Infection, especially viral, e.g. EBV; bacterial, e.g. tuberculosis (TB) (common)
- Chronic lymphocytic leukaemia (CLL): characterised by chronic lymphocytosis, often asymptomatic in its early stages
- Smoking
- Post-splenectomy
- Autoimmune, e.g. RA

History and examination

- Examine for lymphadenopathy and hepatosplenomegaly
- Ask about B symptoms
- Symptoms and signs of infection, autoimmune or connective tissue disorders
- Travel history

Investigations

- Initial:
  - blood film
  - FBC repeat 6 weeks if suspected viral cause (likely to be transient)
- Consider:
  - glandular fever screen
  - autoimmune screen, e.g. ANA, anti-CCP/RF (as per local guidance)

Referral

Emergency admission

- Acutely unwell patient, e.g. with severe infection / sepsis

Urgent suspected cancer

- Suspected haematological malignancy, e.g. abnormal blood film, splenomegaly (haematology)
- Progressive lymphadenopathy (relevant specialty depending upon location)

Urgent outpatient

- Lymphocytosis >30 × 10^9/L (haematology)

Routine outpatient

- Persistent unexplained lymphocytes >5 × 10^9/L (two tests >6 weeks apart), otherwise well (haematology)

High basophils (basophilia) (>0.2 × 10^9/L)

Normal range: 0.0–0.2 × 10^9/L

Background

- Reactive causes are rare: if persistent, particularly >0.4 × 10^9/L, this strongly suggests a myeloproliferative neoplasm

Causes

- Myeloproliferative neoplasms, e.g. CML, myelofibrosis
- Autoimmune, e.g. IBD, hypothyroidism
- Acute illness
- Allergy
- Hyposplenism

History and examination

- Examine for lymphadenopathy and hepatosplenomegaly
- Ask about B symptoms
- Symptoms and signs of infection, autoimmune or connective tissue disorders

Investigations

- Initial:
  - blood film
  - ESR/CRP
  - TFT

Referral

Urgent suspected cancer

- Suspected haematological malignancy, e.g. abnormal blood film, splenomegaly (haematology)

Routine outpatient

- Unexplained persistent basophilia >0.2 × 10^9/L (two tests >6 weeks apart) (haematology)

High eosinophils (eosinophilia) ($>0.5 \times 10^9$/L)

Normal range: $0.04–0.50 \times 10^9$/L

Background

- Eosinophils play a part in allergic, parasitic and malignant disease processes, as well as tissue repair and remodelling
- Hypereosinophilia:
  - defined as eosinophils $>1.5 \times 10^9$/L persisting for >6 months with no obvious cause
  - associated with signs of organ dysfunction:
    - cardiovascular: chest pain, heart failure, venous thromboembolism (VTE)
    - respiratory: dyspnoea, cough and wheeze
    - neurological: cerebrovascular accident (CVA), peripheral neuropathy
    - gastrointestinal: dysphagia, treatment-refractory gastro-oesophageal reflux disease (GORD)

Causes

- Atopy, allergy, e.g. asthma, eczema, rhinitis
- Infections, e.g. parasites, fungal, HIV
- Medication, e.g. angiotensin-converting enzyme inhibitors (ACEi), penicillin, anti-epileptics, proton pump inhibitors (PPIs)
- Gastrointestinal, e.g. chronic pancreatitis, IBD, coeliac
- Respiratory, e.g. asthma, sarcoidosis
- Malignancy, e.g. solid tumours, Hodgkin lymphoma, T-cell non-Hodgkin lymphoma, CML
- Hyposplenism
- Autoimmune, e.g. SLE, RA
- Dermatological, e.g. pemphigoid
- Adrenal insufficiency

History and examination

- Examine for lymphadenopathy and hepatosplenomegaly
- Ask about B symptoms
- Symptoms and signs of infection, autoimmune or connective tissue disorders
- Travel history

Investigations

- Initial:
  - FBC, blood film
  - ESR/CRP
  - vitamin B12 ($\uparrow$ may point to a myeloid disorder)
  - U&E, LFT, bone profile
  - coeliac screen

- Consider:
  - for those with systemic symptoms or persistent eosinophilia $>1.5 \times 10^9$/L, test for causes and evaluate organ damage:
    - autoimmune screen, e.g. ANA, anti-CCP/RF (as per local guidance)
    - parasite investigations, e.g. stool ova cysts, appropriate serology tests
    - CXR: if respiratory symptoms
    - amylase: pancreatic issues
    - hepatitis B and C, HIV

Referral

Emergency admission

- Acutely unwell patient, e.g. with severe infection, or end organ damage

Urgent suspected cancer

- Suspected haematological malignancy, e.g. abnormal blood film, splenomegaly (haematology)
- Suspected malignancy (relevant specialty)

Urgent outpatient

- Eosinophils $>5 \times 10^9$/L without obvious secondary cause (haematology)
- Eosinophils $>1.5 \times 10^9$/L with suspected end organ damage (haematology)

Routine outpatient

- Unexplained persistent eosinophilia $>1.5 \times 10^9$/L (two tests >6 weeks apart), otherwise well (haematology)
- Diagnostic uncertainty (relevant specialty)
- Significant travel history and unsure about appropriate testing (microbiology / infectious diseases)

GP management tips

- For well patients with eosinophilia $0.5-1.5 \times 10^9$/L, further testing may not be indicated
- Unprovoked DVT/PE may be a manifestation of end organ damage

High monocytes (monocytosis)

Normal range: $0.2-1.0 \times 10^9$/L

Background

- This is frequently transient
- Persistent count $>1.0 \times 10^9$/L for >12 months may represent a myeloproliferative disorder (chronic myelomonocytic leukaemia – CMML)

Causes

- Smoking (common cause of mild monocytosis)
- Infections, e.g. TB, malaria
- Autoimmune and inflammatory diseases, e.g. sarcoidosis, RA
- Stress response, e.g. post MI
- Hyposplenism
- CMML (chronic, incurable disorder of varying severity)
- Malignancy

History and examination

- Examine for lymphadenopathy and hepatosplenomegaly
- Ask about B symptoms
- Symptoms and signs of infection, autoimmune or connective tissue disorders

Investigations

- Initial:
  - o blood film
  - o ESR/CRP
  - o U&E, LFT, bone profile
- Consider:
  - o autoimmune screen, e.g. ANA, anti-CCP/RF (as per local guidance)

Referral

Urgent suspected cancer

- Suspected haematological malignancy, e.g. abnormal blood film, splenomegaly (haematology)

Urgent outpatient

- Persistent monocytosis $>5 \times 10^9$/L (two tests >6 weeks apart) (haematology)
- Monocytosis ($1.0–5.0 \times 10^9$/L) with other cytopenia (haematology)

Routine outpatient

- Persistent monocytosis ($1.0–5.0 \times 10^9$/L) (two tests >6 weeks apart), otherwise well (haematology)

2.1.3 Platelets

Low platelets (thrombocytopenia) (platelets $<150 \times 10^9$/L)

Normal range: $150–450 \times 10^9$/L

Background

- Bleeding is rare if platelets $>50 \times 10^9$/L
- Spontaneous bleeding risk increases if $<20 \times 10^9$/L

Causes

- Artefact (platelet clumping)
- Alcohol
- Liver disease
- Pregnancy
- Thyroid dysfunction
- Medication, e.g. NSAIDs, PPI, quinine, digoxin, anti-epileptics, antipsychotics
- Bone marrow failure, e.g. malignant infiltration, myelodysplasia, ↓ B12, ↓ folate
- Infection, e.g. HIV, hepatitis B and C
- Hypersplenism
- Idiopathic thrombocytopenic purpura (ITP)
- Microangiopathic haemolytic anaemias (rarer): disseminated intravascular coagulopathy (DIC), thrombotic thrombocytopenic purpura (TTP), haemolytic uraemic syndrome (HUS)

History and examination

- Examine for lymphadenopathy and hepatosplenomegaly
- Ask about B symptoms
- Symptoms and signs of infection, autoimmune or connective tissue disorders
- Mucocutaneous bleeding, e.g. nose, gums, skin, rectal, vaginal
- Recent infections
- Medication review: anticoagulation, antiplatelets
- Stigmata of liver disease, e.g. spider naevi, ascites

Investigations

- Initial:
  - FBC (if film shows platelet clumps, repeat using citrated sample)
  - B12, folate
  - coagulation screen
  - LFT
  - TFT
- Consider:
  - autoimmune screen, e.g. ANA, anti-CCP/RF (as per local guidance)
  - HIV, hepatitis B and C
  - myeloma screen
  - *H. pylori* testing

Referral

Emergency admission
- Platelets $<20 \times 10^9$/L
- Active bleeding

Urgent outpatient
- Platelets $<50 \times 10^9$/L (haematology)
- Platelets $<80 \times 10^9$/L and associated with any of the following (haematology):
  - other cytopenia (Hb <100 g/L, neutrophils $<1 \times 10^9$/L)
  - splenomegaly, lymphadenopathy
  - forthcoming surgery

Routine outpatient
- Persistent unexplained platelets $<80 \times 10^9$/L (two tests >6 weeks apart) (haematology)
- History of thrombosis (haematology)
- Liver disease (hepatology)
- Platelets $>80 \times 10^9$/L: if no cause found (haematology) – may require interval monitoring and referral if things change

GP management tips

- Consider stopping all antiplatelet agents and anticoagulation if platelets $<50 \times 10^9$/L

High platelets (thrombocytosis) (platelets $>450 \times 10^9$/L)

Normal range: $150–450 \times 10^9$/L

Background

- Patients can develop thrombosis or bleeding due to abnormal platelet function

Causes

- Secondary (commoner):
  - infection, inflammation
  - medication, e.g. steroids
  - bleeding, iron deficiency
  - surgery, trauma
  - hyposplenism or previous splenectomy
  - connective tissue disorders, e.g. RA
  - malignancy
- Primary (rarer): more suggestive if there is an accompanying erythrocytosis or leucocytosis, arterial or venous thrombotic events, or abnormal bleeding
  - myeloproliferative disorders, e.g. essential thrombocythaemia, CML, polycythaemia vera, myelofibrosis

History and examination

- Examine for lymphadenopathy and hepatosplenomegaly
- Ask about B symptoms
- Symptoms and signs of infection, autoimmune or connective tissue disorders
- Bleeding or risk factors for iron-deficiency anaemia
- Consider red flag symptoms of malignancy

Investigations

- Initial:
  - blood film
  - ESR/CRP
  - ferritin, iron studies
  - U&E, LFT, bone profile
- Consider
  - autoimmune screen, e.g. ANA, anti-CCP/RF (as per local guidance)
  - investigation for occult malignancy as appropriate:
    - CXR: age ≥40 years within 2 weeks (lung cancer)
    - pelvis USS: visible haematuria or vaginal discharge (unexplained) in women age ≥55 years (endometrial cancer)
    - FIT (colorectal cancer)
    - non-urgent direct access OGD: age ≥55 with nausea / vomiting / ↓ weight / reflux / dyspepsia / upper abdominal pain (oesophageal or stomach cancer)

Referral

Emergency admission

- Neurological symptoms
- Active bleeding

Urgent outpatient

- Unexplained thrombocytosis >1000 × 10^9/L (haematology)
- Thrombocytosis with history of the following (haematology):
  - recent (last 3 months) arterial or venous thromboembolism (including DVT/PE, CVA/TIA, peripheral vascular disease, MI / unstable angina)
  - associated abnormal FBC indices

Routine outpatient

- Persistent unexplained thrombocytosis (two tests >6 weeks apart) (haematology)

GP management tips

- ↑ inflammation markers?
  - likely reactive thrombocytosis; treat as appropriate and monitor response
- Iron deficiency?
  - treat as appropriate and monitor response

2.2 Reticulocytes

Normal range: 0.5–2.5% or 40–100 × 10⁹/L

Background

- Reticulocytes are an important index of effective erythropoiesis
- They help differentiate between a red cell production problem versus increased consumption or loss:
  - anaemia without ↑ reticulocytes – indicates ↓ production of reticulocytes, i.e. an inadequate response to correct the anaemia
  - anaemia with ↑ reticulocytes – indicates loss of red blood cells, e.g. from haemolysis or bleeding, with ↑ compensatory production of reticulocytes

Causes

- ↓ reticulocytes:
  - ↓ iron, B12 and folate
  - anaemia of chronic disease
  - aplastic anaemia
  - myelodysplastic syndromes
- ↑ reticulocytes:
  - haemolytic anaemia
  - blood loss
  - response to therapy, e.g. iron, folate, B12 (↑ reticulocytes is the earliest sign of a positive response to replacement therapy)

History and examination

- Consider the reason for testing and the above causes
- Note, test may be part of work-up for suspected Gilbert's syndrome (Hb, reticulocytes and blood film normal)

Investigations

- Initial:
  - FBC, blood film
  - B12, folate, ferritin/iron studies
  - U&E, LFT
- Consider:
  - haemolysis screen
    - ↑ LDH, ↑ bilirubin, ↑ reticulocytes are consistent with haemolysis
    - blood film and direct Coombs' test (DCT) will help distinguish the type

Referral

Routine outpatient

- Suspected haemolysis (haematology); urgency dependent on clinical judgement

2.3 Immunoglobulins / serum protein electrophoresis / serum free light chains / urine Bence Jones proteins

Normal ranges

- Immunoglobulins (Ig):
  - IgG: 5.8–15.4 g/L
  - IgA: 0.64–2.97 g/L
  - IgM (♂): 0.24–1.90 g/L
  - IgM (♀): 0.75–2.30 g/L
- Electrophoresis: qualitative report given (e.g. monoclonal, polyclonal)
- Paraprotein: 0 g/L
- Kappa (K) light chain: 3.3–19.4 mg/L
- Lambda (λ) light chain: 5.71–26.30 mg/L
- Serum free light chain (sFLC) ratio (K/λ):   0.26–1.65 (if normal renal function, eGFR ≥60 mL/min)
       0.37–3.10 (if renal impairment, eGFR <60 mL/min)
- Urine Bence Jones proteins (BJP):   nil

Background

Immunoglobulins

- Checks absolute levels of immunoglobulins IgA, IgG and IgM
- Immunoglobulins are proteins consisting of 2 heavy and 2 light chains produced by terminally differentiated B cells (or plasma cells) that are important in immunity
- There are 5 classes of Ig in normal serum determined by their heavy chains: 80% is IgG, 15% IgA, 5% IgM, 0.2% IgD, with trace IgE
- Levels are age- and sex-dependent

Paraproteins (monoclonal proteins or M-bands)

- Abnormal Ig produced by clonal plasma cells
- Detected on serum electrophoresis (and immunofixation reflexed by the lab)
- Paraproteins have various causes that vary in their clinical significance:
  - malignant B-cell disorders:
    - multiple myeloma
    - plasmacytoma (solitary or extramedullary)
    - lymphoproliferative disorders, e.g. CLL, non-Hodgkin lymphomas including Waldenström's macroglobulinaemia
    - amyloidosis (large tongue, unexplained heart failure, peripheral neuropathy, carpal tunnel syndrome or nephrotic syndrome)
  - monoclonal gammopathy of unknown significance (MGUS): paraprotein

detected with no evidence of other B-cell disorder
- o non-malignant systemic disease:
  - ▪ infection, e.g. TB, endocarditis
  - ▪ autoimmune disease, e.g. RA, scleroderma
  - ▪ liver disease
  - ▪ cutaneous disease, e.g. pyoderma gangrenosum

Serum free light chains (sFLC)

- Light chains assayed in serum
- Preferred method of checking light chains
- Has replaced urine Bence Jones proteins in some areas – check local lab guidance
- The 2 isotypes of light chains are kappa (K) and lambda (λ)

Urine Bence Jones proteins (BJP)

- Light chains detected in urine
- Has been replaced by sFLC in some areas – check local lab guidance

Indication for testing

- Suspected monoclonal B-cell lymphoproliferative disease, e.g. myeloma, lymphoma or CLL
  - o immunoglobulins, protein electrophoresis and free light chain assessment (by checking urine Bence Jones proteins or serum free light chains) should all be tested together to assess for paraprotein and associated suppression of normal immunoglobulins
  - o serial monitoring can be used to assess disease progression, e.g. with MGUS
- Assessing conditions with ↑ globulins, e.g.
  - o connective tissue disease
  - o chronic liver disease
  - o chronic infection: untreated HIV

Interpretation

Immunoglobulins

- Depending upon the clinical condition, levels of the different Ig may be ↑ or ↓, or there may be a combined picture with ↑ in certain classes and ↓ in others
- Measurement of serum Ig does not provide categorical diagnosis of any disease
- ↑ Ig does not necessarily mean there is a paraprotein (commonest cause is inflammation or infection)
- Normal levels do not exclude a small paraprotein

Paraproteins (monoclonal proteins or M-bands)

- Serum electrophoresis is required to determine whether an ↑ Ig level is monoclonal or polyclonal
  - o if a monoclonal Ig is identified, immunofixation is reflexed by the lab to type the monoclonal protein

o   serum Ig **must** be accompanied by serum electrophoresis and free light chain assessment (sFLC, **or** urine BJP, if sFLC are not available) to look for paraproteins
- If no monoclonal protein is identified on serum electrophoresis and urine / serum free light chain assessment is normal, $\uparrow$ Ig is polyclonal

Serum free light chains (sFLC)

- Normally secreted by bone marrow plasma cells in a 2:1 ratio of K:λ
- λ chains are excreted more slowly by the kidney, so the sFLC ratio is normally close to 1:1
- It is normal to have more serum K light chains than λ
- Renal impairment impairs excretion of both isotypes, so the sFLC ratio can be 0.37–3.10 if eGFR <60 mL/min
- In an acute phase response, both λ and K may be $\uparrow$, giving a normal ratio
- A sFLC falling significantly outside of the normal range implies a clonal B-cell disorder: myeloma causes an abnormal ratio and high absolute levels of either K or λ
- Abnormal ratios close to the normal range are more difficult to interpret and may be benign

Urine Bence Jones proteins (BJP)

- If positive, this means light chains have been detected
- Request sFLC if available

GP management tips

- A complete myeloma screen involves requesting Ig, serum electrophoresis and assessing free light chains (via sFLC **or** urine BJP, if sFLC are not available)
- Do not use serum protein electrophoresis, serum immunofixation, sFLC or urine BJP alone to exclude a diagnosis of myeloma
- Referrals to haematology should *only* be made if there are monoclonal paraproteins on serum electrophoresis, an abnormal sFLC ratio, or positive urine BJP. Myeloma is unlikely if:
  o   normal Ig levels
  o   no serum paraprotein
  o   normal sFLC ratio
  o   no BJP
- Polyclonal hypergammaglobulinaemia is not associated with underlying haematological disorders: it implies a non-specific immune reaction, e.g. due to infection, inflammation or neoplasia
- With hypogammaglobulinaemia, ensure full myeloma screen is completed and look for signs of lymphoma (e.g. check for lymphocytosis, exclude lymphadenopathy)
- Multiple banding:
  o   often seen in inflammatory conditions: investigate possible causes
  o   repeat in 4–6 months to ensure no larger band appears
  o   if still present and cause unknown, refer haematology

- Possible band:
  - o repeat in 4–6 months to ensure no larger band appears
  - o if a possible band is persistent then refer for haematology advice and guidance, as may need MGUS assessment
- Referral criteria:
  - o emergency admission
    - acutely unwell, e.g. acute kidney injury, significant hypercalcaemia or spinal cord compression
  - o urgent suspected cancer (haematology)
    - moderate concentration of paraprotein, e.g. IgG >15 g/L, IgM or IgA >10 g/L
    - identification of IgD or IgE paraprotein (regardless of concentration)
    - significantly abnormal sFLC ratio (<0.1 or >7) or identification of BJP
    - any serum paraprotein <10 g/L but where there is clinical suspicion of myeloma
    - imaging confirming a lytic bone lesion or abnormality suspicious of myeloma
  - o routine (haematology)
    - if minor levels of paraprotein (IgG <15 g/L, IgA or IgM <10 g/L) or mildly abnormal sFLC ratio (>0.1 or <7, but outside normal range) without symptoms of myeloma
      - recheck the serum or urine in 2–3 months to monitor the disease pattern
      - if paraprotein concentration ↑ by >25% and >5 g/L or if symptoms develop, make urgent haematology referral
    - diagnostic uncertainty

2.4 Clotting tests

Coagulation screen

Normal values:	
Prothrombin time (PT):	9–13 sec
Activated partial thromboplastin time (APTT):	22–36 sec
Fibrinogen:	1.5–4.5 g/L

Background

- Useful to screen for bleeding disorders in those with a suggestive bleeding history:
  - o bleeding associated with trauma or surgery, e.g. dental procedures (was there abnormal bleeding, a transfusion required, or additional intervention to achieve haemostasis?)
  - o heavy menstrual bleeding from menarche
  - o bleeding around pregnancy or delivery
  - o bruising or excess bleeding in minor injuries
  - o spontaneous bleeding: gastrointestinal, joint/muscle bleeds, intracranial haemorrhage, epistaxis

- An abnormal screen does not necessarily indicate an increase in the risk of bleeding
- A normal screen does not rule out a bleeding disorder
- Bleeding disorders with normal coagulation screen include:
  - von Willebrand's disease
  - platelet function defects
  - medication, e.g. antiplatelets, apixaban
  - mild factor deficiency
  - connective tissue disorders, e.g. Ehlers–Danlos
  - vitamin C deficiency
  - hereditary haemorrhagic telangiectasia
  - uraemia

Indications for testing

- Before starting anticoagulation
- Investigating thrombocytopenia
- To look for a lupus anticoagulant
- Monitor anticoagulant (only with specific assay, e.g. international normalised ratio (INR) for warfarin)
- A bleeding history
- Monitor severity of liver disease

Interpretation

- Prolonged PT:
  - warfarin
  - liver disease
  - vitamin K deficiency
  - factor deficiency, e.g. VII (rare)
- Prolonged APTT:
  - warfarin
  - liver disease
- Vitamin K deficiency:
  - antiphospholipid antibodies: despite being a disorder that causes clots, this occurs due to the assay interference (look for lab comments, as they will reflex further tests)
  - factor deficiency:
    - haemophilia A (VIII)
    - haemophilia B (IX)
    - haemophilia C (XI)
    - von Willebrand's disease (vWF pairs up with factor VIII)
- Prolonged PT and APTT:
  - liver disease
  - warfarin
  - vitamin K deficiency
  - inherited deficiencies of factors II, V and X

- Fibrinogen (factor I) is an acute phase reactant:
  - o increases in:
    - inflammation/infection
    - tissue damage, e.g. MI, trauma, stroke
    - malignancy
  - o decreases in:
    - inherited deficiency
    - liver disease
    - malnutrition

Referral

Emergency admission

- Active bleeding

Urgent outpatient

- Unexplained abnormal coagulation screen (haematology)

Routine outpatient

- Liver abnormality (hepatology)
- Suggestive personal or family history of bleeding disorder, even if coagulation normal (haematology)

2.5 Blood film comments

Follow any advice accompanying blood film reports

Findings	Differential diagnosis
Anisocytosis (variation in size)	Megaloblastic anaemia, IDA, thalassaemia
Basophilic stippling	Thalassaemia traits
Bite cells (degmacytes)	G6PD deficiency, oxidative stress, unstable haemoglobins
Blast cells	Myelofibrosis, leukaemia
Burr cells (echinocytes, crenated red cells)	Artifact, uraemia, malnutrition
Dimorphic red cells	Two populations, e.g. iron deficiency responding to iron, mixed iron and B12 or folate deficiencies
Elliptocytes	Hereditary elliptocytosis (>25%)
Fragmented red cells (schistocytes, helmet cells, keratocytes)	Thrombotic micro-angiopathic haemolytic anaemias, e.g. TTP, HUS
Heinz bodies	G6PD deficiency
Howell–Jolly bodies (nuclear remnants)	Splenectomy, rarely in leukaemia, megaloblastic anaemia, IDA

Findings	Differential diagnosis
Hyper-segmented neutrophil nuclei	Megaloblastic anaemia, uraemia, liver disease
Hypochromic red cells	Reduced Hb synthesis, e.g. iron deficiency, thalassaemia
Increased reticulocytes	Bleeding, haemolysis, marrow infiltration, severe hypoxia, response to haematinic therapy
Irreversibly sickled red cells (drepanocytes)	Sickle cell syndromes (SS, SC, Sβ-thalassaemia)
Macrocytic red cells	Alcohol/liver disease, myelodysplastic syndrome (MDS), compensated haemolysis, B12 or folate deficiency, hypothyroidism, chronic respiratory failure, aplastic anaemia
Microcytic red cells	Iron deficiency, thalassaemia
Oval macrocytes	Megaloblastic anaemia, IDA, thalassaemia
Pencil cells	Iron deficiency
Poikilocytosis (variation in shape)	Megaloblastic anaemia, IDA, acute haemolytic anaemia
Polychromasia (uneven staining)	Caused by younger red blood cells staining blue, e.g. bleeding, haemolysis, iron and B12 replacement
Rouleaux	Chronic inflammation, paraproteinaemia, myeloma
Schistocytes (fragment of red blood cells)	Intravascular haemolysis
Sideroblasts (normoblasts with stainable iron)	Haemolytic anaemia, megaloblastic anaemia, haemochromatosis
Spherocytes	Autoimmune haemolysis, hereditary spherocytosis
Spur cells (acanthocytes)	Liver disease, renal failure
Stomatocytes	Artifact, liver disease, alcoholism, obstructive lung disease
Target cells	Liver disease, thalassaemia, sickle cell disease and occasionally IDA
Teardrop cells (dacrocytes)	Marrow infiltrations, hereditary elliptocytosis, severe iron deficiency, megaloblastic anaemia, thalassaemia

Adapted from: Adewoyin, A.S. and Nwogoh, B. (2014) Peripheral blood film – a review. *Ann Ib Postgrad Med,* **12**: 71 and Provan, D. (ed.) (2018) *Oxford Handbook of Clinical and Laboratory Investigation,* 4th ed. Oxford.

2.6 Inflammatory markers: CRP/ESR/PV

C-reactive protein (CRP) normal range: <10 mg/L

Erythrocyte sedimentation rate (ESR) normal range: ♂ 0–22 mm/h; ♀ 0–29 mm/h

Plasma viscosity (PV) normal range: 1.50–1.72 mPa.s

Background

- Non-specific tests of inflammation/infection
- Request and interpret as per the clinical context
- False ↑ ESR: anaemia or delay in sample transport
- CRP is more sensitive and rapidly responding than ESR
- CRP: acute phase protein, so elevated in infection (especially bacterial vs. viral), often normal in malignancy
- ESR is more useful than CRP in the following: suspected polymyalgia rheumatica (PMR), giant cell arteritis (GCA), SLE, vasculitis, IBD and exclusion of osteomyelitis in diabetic foot ulcers
- Causes of ↑ levels:
  - infection
  - inflammation: autoimmune disease, e.g. PMR, sarcoidosis
  - malignancy: myeloma, lymphoma
  - ↑ immunoglobulins
  - trauma
  - smoking
  - obesity
  - pregnancy

Indication for testing

- Suspected infection, inflammation or neoplasia
  - note these markers are non-specific
    - obesity causes ↑ CRP
    - ESR ↑ with age
    - PV is independent of age, sex, and Hb
- Monitoring disease activity and response to treatment, e.g. infection

Interpretation

- Check lab guidance for preferred inflammatory marker tests locally
- Normal inflammatory markers do not exclude disease: use clinical judgement and refer if concerns
- Testing multiple inflammatory markers does not improve the ability to rule out disease, but does increase the risk that at least one of the tests will give a false positive
- The overall diagnostic utility of all three inflammatory markers is similar and low
  - CRP marginally outperforms ESR and PV for infections (changes more rapidly)
  - CRP tends to be cheaper than ESR and PV
- Thus, CRP should generally be the 1st-line test, except in myeloma: ESR and PV are superior to CRP, but other relevant tests are needed if suspected (immunoglobulins, serum electrophoresis and free light chain assessment (sFLC, or urine BJP if sFLC not available))

What test should be used?

Scenario	CRP	ESR	PV	Comments
Acute infection	Y	N	N	CRP changes most rapidly
Suspected myeloma?	N	Y	Y	NICE advises ESR or PV
				If suspected, check the appropriate bloods: immunoglobulins, serum electrophoresis and free light chain assessment (sFLC, or urine BJP if sFLC not available)

2.7 Iron studies and ferritin

2.7.1 Iron studies

Background

This includes the following tests:
- *Ferritin:*
  - the intracellular storage form of iron
  - an acute phase protein: $\uparrow$ in inflammation, liver disease and malignancy; in these patients, ferritin can appear either falsely $\uparrow$ or normal, when stores are $\downarrow$
  - levels $\downarrow$ in iron deficiency (in the absence of inflammation)
- *Serum iron:*
  - ferric ions (Fe^{3+}) bound to serum transferrin
  - affected by dietary iron intake, inflammation and infection
- *Transferrin:*
  - main iron transport protein in plasma
  - $\uparrow$ in iron deficiency
  - $\downarrow$ in iron overload
  - total iron-binding capacity (TIBC) is an alternative test, reflecting the availability of iron-binding sites on transferrin; levels will vary as per transferrin
- *Transferrin saturation:*
  - calculated from serum iron and either TIBC or transferrin
  - $\uparrow$ in iron overload
  - $\downarrow$ in iron deficiency
  - does not quantitatively reflect iron stores: $\uparrow$ with dietary iron; wait 4 weeks after cessation of treatment before requesting iron studies

Indications for testing

- Suspected iron overload:
  - symptoms
    - early: may be asymptomatic or present with vague symptoms, e.g. fatigue, weakness or generalised joint pains
    - later: deranged LFTs, cirrhosis, erectile dysfunction, arthritis or cardiomyopathy

- o causes
  - ■ primary: haemochromatosis
  - ■ secondary: iron supplements, repeat blood transfusions, iron-loading anaemias (e.g. chronic haemolytic anaemia, beta-thalassaemia)
- Suspected iron deficiency:
  - o investigating aetiology of anaemia
  - o malabsorption, e.g. investigation of unintentional weight loss or chronic diarrhoea, coeliac disease, post-surgery, e.g. gastrectomy
  - o bleeding, e.g. menstruation, GI, renal tract
  - o functional iron deficiency, i.e. there are adequate iron stores which are inadequately utilised, e.g. chronic kidney disease (CKD), malignancy
- Response to treatment, e.g. iron therapy

Interpretation

Test	Scenario				
	Iron deficiency without anaemia	IDA	Anaemia of chronic disease	IDA and anaemia of chronic disease	Iron overload
Haemoglobin Adult ♂: <130 g/L Adult ♀: <115 g/L	N	↓	↓	↓	N
MCV: 80–100 fL	N or ↓	↓	N or mildly ↓	↓	N
Ferritin Premenopausal women: 15–200 µg/L Men and postmenopausal women: 20–300 µg/L	↓	↓	N or ↑	N or ↓	↑
Transferrin: 2.0–3.5 g/L *or* **TIBC:** 45–81 µmol/L	N or ↑	↑	N or ↓	N or ↑	↓
Serum iron: 10–30 nmol/L	↓	↓	↓	↓	↑
Transferrin saturation: 25–45%	N or ↓	↓	N or ↓	↓	↑

GP management tips

- Check if on iron supplements, prescribed or over the counter (OTC)
- Iron overload typically results in ↑ ferritin and ↑ transferrin saturation
- Iron deficiency is best assessed using serum ferritin, which is ↓ in the absence of infection or inflammation
- Ferritin levels can be ↑ by inflammatory processes and can mask iron deficiency

- If ↑ transferrin saturation is the only biochemical abnormality or the result is borderline, repeat the test on a fasting sample to eliminate any rise caused by dietary iron
- ↑ iron, ↑ transferrin saturation, and ↑ ferritin can be seen in acute hepatic injury due to leakage of intracellular contents and can incorrectly give the impression of iron overload
- A raised ferritin is **not** specific for haemochromatosis; check for ↑ transferrin saturation

2.7.2 Ferritin

Normal range: ♂: 12–300 µg/L   ♀: 10–200 µg/L

Indications for testing

- Assess and monitor iron deficiency
- Monitor response to iron therapy
- Differentiate iron deficiency from chronic disease as a cause of anaemia
- Assess for iron overload
- Assessing restless legs syndrome, fibromyalgia symptoms

Interpretation

- ↑ ferritin levels are found in:
  - acute and chronic liver disease
  - infection
  - inflammation
  - alcoholism
  - malignancy
  - hyperthyroidism
  - iron overload, e.g. haemochromatosis
  - end-stage renal disease
  - anaemia of chronic disease
- ↓ ferritin levels are found in:
  - iron deficiency (with or without anaemia), e.g. due to inadequate dietary intake, increased body needs, reduced absorption, chronic inflammation and chronic blood loss
  - haemodialysis

GP management tips

Assessing raised ferritin levels (♂ >300 µg/L; ♀ >200 µg/L)

Background

- Identifying the cause is important to exclude serious pathology as well as to prevent potential organ-specific complications
- A raised ferritin is **not** specific for haemochromatosis

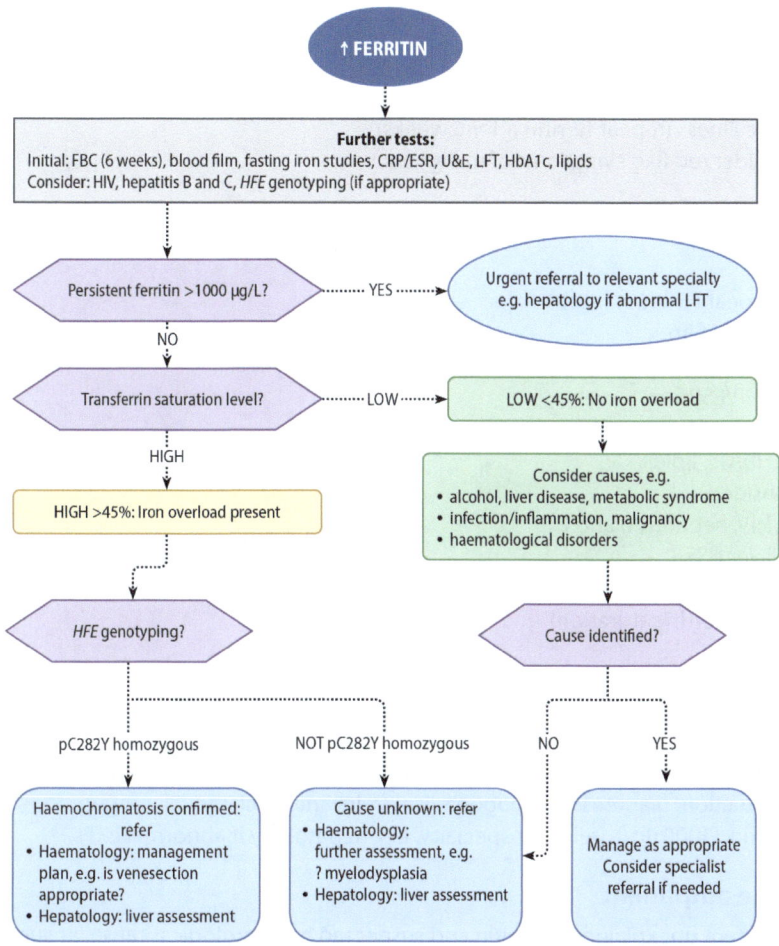

Causes

- Hereditary haemochromatosis: autosomal recessive condition caused by mutation of the *HFE* gene. Pathological iron overload may affect the liver, pancreas, heart, pituitary gland and joints
- Liver disease: hepatitis, metabolic syndrome, diabetes
- Lifestyle causes: alcohol and smoking
- Infection, inflammation (repeat ferritin 6 weeks after illness to ensure resolution)
- Malignancy
- Autoimmune disease
- Renal failure
- Chronic blood transfusion / IV iron therapy
- Thalassaemia (even without blood transfusion)
- Myelodysplasia

History and examination

- Alcohol, liver disease
- FHx
- Acute illness (repeat ferritin after 6 weeks)
- Consider red flag symptoms of malignancy

Investigations

- Initial:
  - repeat FBC (6 weeks)
  - blood film
  - fasting iron studies (eliminates dietary iron influence)
  - CRP/ESR
  - U&E, LFT
  - HbA1c, lipids
- Consider:
  - HIV, hepatitis B and C
  - liver USS
  - *HFE* genotyping (test if a positive FHx of haemochromatosis or ↑ ferritin and ↓ transferrin saturation)

Referral

Urgent outpatient

- ↑ ferritin with evidence of unexplained end-organ damage, e.g. heart failure, liver dysfunction, diabetes or hypogonadism (relevant specialty)
- Ferritin >1000 µg/L (relevant specialty, e.g. hepatology if abnormal LFT)

Routine outpatient

- Persistent unexplained ↑ ferritin and suspected haematological cause (as suggested by blood film or count), e.g. thalassaemia, transfusion overload, inherited anaemia or myelodysplasia (haematology)
- Confirmed homozygous pC282Y (which confirms haemochromatosis) for management advice (haematology, hepatology)
- Genetic counselling for confirmed haemochromatosis (genetics)

References

References to support all aspects of testing and management guidance can be found, broken up by section, by scanning the QR code below or clicking on the Resources tab on the page for this book at www.scionpublishing.com/lab_results

Chapter 3

Immunology and rheumatology

Follow your local reference ranges, clinical pathways, management and referral guidance. This guidance is not a substitute for individual clinical judgement. Reference ranges will vary according to the assay used by laboratories. Those provided are examples and may vary in your locality.

3.1 Immunology (autoantibodies)

3.1.1 Statistics definitions

	Disease present	Disease absent
Positive test	True positive	False positive
Negative test	False negative	True negative

- Sensitivity: the proportion of people with a disease with a positive test
  Sensitivity = true positives / (true positives + false negatives)
- Specificity: the proportion of people without a disease with a negative test
  Specificity = true negatives / (true negatives + false positives)
- Positive predictive value (PPV): the proportion of people with a positive test who actually have the disease
  PPV = true positives / (true positives + false positives)
- Negative predictive value (NPV): the proportion of people with a negative test who actually do not have the disease
  NPV = true negatives / (true negatives + false negatives)

Background

- These test for antibodies against specific antigens
- Useful for diagnostic, prognostic and disease monitoring purposes
- Tests must be interpreted considering the clinical context:
  - they are often not specific to one disease
  - tests may be positive in healthy individuals
  - refer if clinical concern despite normal tests or if diagnostic uncertainty
- Avoid requesting tests indiscriminately for non-specific symptoms as they have a low PPV, i.e. if the tests are performed on patients with no real clinical evidence of relevant disease, most of the positive results will be found in patients without disease
- Most autoantibodies are measured using immunoassays, e.g. enzyme-linked immunosorbent assay (ELISA)
  - results are reported as a titre, e.g. 1:80, or in standardised international units (IU/mL)
- Positivity of certain autoantibodies in low titres, e.g. 1:40, in the absence of relevant clinical features, have little consequence
  - generally, the higher the reported titre, the more likely that there is an associated illness, with definite positivity ≥1:640

3.1.2 Antinuclear antibodies (ANA)

Normal: ANA negative; clinically significant titres of ANA are usually >1:160

- Indication for testing: suspected connective tissue disease (CTD), autoimmune liver disease
- **Not** useful for disease monitoring, and rarely need to be repeated after diagnosis
- Results may be reported in two components: titre and staining pattern

Titre

- This is the quantity of ANA in the serum: the higher the titre, the more likely will be the diagnosis of CTD, with definite positivity ≥1:640
- ↑ titres found in (sensitivity in brackets):
  - rheumatic conditions:
    - systemic lupus erythematosus (SLE) (93%)
    - systemic sclerosis (85%)
    - Sjögren's syndrome (44%)
    - polymyositis / dermatomyositis (61%)
    - rheumatoid arthritis (RA) (41%)
  - infection, e.g. endocarditis, tuberculosis (TB), infectious mononucleosis
  - inflammation, e.g. autoimmune hepatitis, primary biliary cholangitis (PBC), Crohn's
  - malignancy
  - medication, e.g. phenytoin, tetracyclines, terbinafine
  - healthy people – ANA 1:160 occur in 5% of healthy individuals
- Low titre ANA is common, especially with infections and in the elderly
  - in people aged >70, up to 70% have a positive ANA of 1:40
- Labs will likely reflex further tests if ANA titres are above a certain threshold, e.g. >1:320, ENA and dsDNA antibodies may be tested

Staining pattern

- This is the pattern of antibody binding to the nucleus
- As there are overlapping disease entities and more specific autoantibodies available, the emphasis on staining pattern in diagnoses has diminished
- Patterns associated with different diseases are:
  - homogeneous: SLE, mixed CTD, drug-induced lupus, RA
  - speckled: SLE, Sjögren's, polymyositis, dermatomyositis, systemic sclerosis
  - nucleolar: diffuse systemic sclerosis, polymyositis
  - centromere: limited systemic sclerosis – CREST (Calcinosis, Raynaud's, oEsophageal dysmotility, Sclerodactyly, Telangiectasia) syndrome
  - peripheral (rim): SLE, systemic sclerosis

3.1.3 Cyclic citrullinated peptide antibodies (CCP)

Normal: negative

- Indication for testing: suspected RA (but **not** pathognomonic)
  - NICE specifies for suspected RA:
    - investigations should not delay referral for specialist opinion
    - offer rheumatoid factor (RF) first
    - consider anti-CCP if negative for RF
- Check your local lab protocols for anti-CCP vs. RF test requests – some labs are moving towards stopping RF requests from primary care in preference of anti-CCP
- Anti-CCP is considered more useful than RF as it:
  - has better sensitivity and specificity than RF
  - appears earlier than RF
  - is unaffected by treatment
  - predicts the development of erosions
- Present in 2% of healthy individuals

3.1.4 Double-stranded DNA antibodies (dsDNA)

Normal: negative

- Indication for testing: suspected SLE, autoimmune liver disease
  - if ANA is strongly positive, e.g. >1/320, the lab will automatically test dsDNA
- Highly specific for SLE (~99%)
- Present in 1% of healthy individuals
- Useful for monitoring disease activity, so test may be repeated over the disease course
- Labs may use different testing methods to test dsDNA antibodies, e.g. ELISA, *Crithidia luciliae* immunofluorescence assay (CLIFT), and radioimmunoassay methods; if antibody tests are associated with positive *Crithidia* staining, then they are more specific

3.1.5 Endomysial antibodies

Normal: negative

- Indication for testing: suspected coeliac disease, but not 1st-line according to NICE
- Ensure gluten-containing foods are eaten in more than one meal a day, for a minimum of 6 weeks before testing
- Check your local lab protocols for coeliac disease serological testing
  - NICE advises labs use:
    - 1st-line: total IgA and IgA tissue transglutaminase (tTG)
    - 2nd-line: IgA endomysial antibodies (EMA) if IgA tTGA testing is unavailable or IgA tTG is weakly positive
    - if IgA deficient (total IgA <0.07 g/L): IgG EMA, IgG deamidated gliadin peptide (DGP) or IgG tTG can be checked

3.1.6 Extractable nuclear antigen antibodies (ENA)

Normal: negative

- Indication for testing: suspected connective tissue disease
  - if ANA is strongly positive, e.g. >1/320, the lab will automatically test anti-ENA, so this does not need to be specifically requested from primary care
- **Not** useful for disease monitoring, and rarely need to be repeated after diagnosis
- Each have their disease associations (not likely to be requested directly from primary care but may be a reflex result from the lab):
  - anti-centromere: limited cutaneous systemic sclerosis, PBC
  - anti-Ro (SS-A): SLE, Sjögren's, neonatal lupus, congenital heart block
  - anti-La (SS-B): SLE, Sjögren's, neonatal lupus, congenital heart block
  - anti-Sm: SLE, lupus nephritis
  - anti-RNP: SLE, mixed CTD (in absence of Sm)
  - anti-Scl 70: generalised scleroderma
  - anti-Jo-1: polymyositis
  - anti-ribosomal P: SLE with psychiatric symptoms
  - anti-chromatin: SLE with nephritis
  - anti-dsDNA: SLE
  - anti-histone: drug-induced lupus

3.1.7 Gastric parietal cell antibodies

Normal: negative

- Indication for testing: suspected pernicious anaemia, autoimmune gastritis (2nd-line according to NICE after intrinsic factor antibody if autoimmune gastritis is still suspected despite a negative intrinsic factor antibody test)
- NICE advises:
  - 1st-line test for suspected autoimmune gastritis in those with vitamin B12 deficiency: anti-intrinsic factor antibody test if not had a positive test for this at any time **or** an operation that could affect vitamin B12 absorption, e.g. total gastrectomy or complete terminal ileal resection
  - when interpreting anti-intrinsic factor antibody test results:
    - follow guidance provided by the lab
    - be aware that a negative test result does not rule out the presence of autoimmune gastritis
  - 2nd-line: an anti-gastric parietal cell antibody test
    - if autoimmune gastritis is still suspected despite a negative anti-intrinsic factor antibody test
- High degree of sensitivity (90%) but poor specificity, especially in the elderly
- Present in other autoimmune diseases too, e.g. autoimmune thyroiditis, type 1 diabetes, Addison's disease
- Present in 5% of healthy individuals, rising to 16% of women aged >60

3.1.8 Intrinsic factor antibodies

Normal: negative

- Indication for testing: suspected pernicious anaemia, autoimmune gastritis (1st-line according to NICE)
- NICE advises:
  - 1st-line test for suspected autoimmune gastritis in those with vitamin B12 deficiency: anti-intrinsic factor antibody test if not had a positive test for this at any time **or** an operation that could affect vitamin B12 absorption, e.g. total gastrectomy or complete terminal ileal resection
  - when interpreting anti-intrinsic factor antibody test results:
    - follow guidance provided by the lab
    - be aware that a negative test result does not rule out the presence of autoimmune gastritis
  - 2nd-line: an anti-gastric parietal cell antibody test
    - if autoimmune gastritis is still suspected despite a negative anti-intrinsic factor antibody test
- Very specific for pernicious anaemia, but poor sensitivity (only present in 50–70% of people with the condition)
- Present in other autoimmune diseases too, e.g. autoimmune thyroiditis, type 1 diabetes

3.1.9 Antimitochondrial antibodies (AMA)

Normal: negative

- Indication for testing: suspected PBC (usually requested as part of autoimmune liver screen in abnormal LFTs)
- Highly sensitive and specific for PBC
- Less commonly found in other autoimmune liver diseases, thyroid disease, SLE

3.1.10 Rheumatoid factor (RF)

Normal range: <20 IU/mL

- Indication for testing: suspected RA (but **not** pathognomonic)
  - NICE specifies for suspected RA:
    - investigations should not delay referral for specialist opinion
    - offer RF first
    - consider anti-CCP if negative for RF
- Check your local lab protocols for anti-CCP vs. RF test requests – some labs are moving towards stopping RF requests from primary care in preference of anti-CCP
- Useful for secondary care use in guiding prognosis (high levels are associated with complications such as systemic symptoms and more severe disease)
- Absent in 30–40% of patients with RA, especially in early disease
- Present in 2% of healthy individuals
- Also present in:
  - autoimmune disease, e.g. Sjögren's syndrome, SLE, PBC, sarcoidosis
  - infections, e.g. bacterial (endocarditis, TB), viral (HIV, hepatitis B/C)

3.1.11 Smooth muscle antibodies

Normal: negative

- Indication for testing: suspected autoimmune liver disease (usually part of liver screen for abnormal LFTs)
- Also present in PBC, CTD and infections, e.g. acute viral hepatitis, infectious mononucleosis
- Low titres are common; found in <2% of the normal population

3.1.12 Tissue transglutaminase (tTG) antibodies

Normal: negative

- Indication for testing: suspected coeliac disease; 1st-line according to NICE
- Highly specific and sensitive test
- Ensure gluten-containing foods are eaten in more than one meal a day, for a minimum of 6 weeks before testing
- Check your local lab protocols for coeliac disease serological testing
  - NICE advises labs use:
    - 1st-line: total IgA and IgA tTG
    - 2nd-line: IgA endomysial antibodies (EMA) if IgA tTGA testing is unavailable or IgA tTG is weakly positive
    - if IgA deficient (total IgA <0.07 g/L): IgG EMA, IgG deamidated gliadin peptide (DGP) or IgG tTG can be checked

3.1.13 Thyroid antibodies

Thyroid peroxidase antibodies (TPO)

Normal: negative

- Indication for testing:
  - primary hypothyroidism (positive in autoimmune thyroid disease)
  - suspected subclinical hypothyroidism (positive result can predict progression to overt hypothyroidism)
- Serial measurements are not helpful

3.2 Immunochemistry

3.2.1 Serum immunoglobulins (Ig), protein electrophoresis

Ig normal range:
- IgG: 5.8–15.4 g/L
- IgA: 0.64–2.97 g/L
- IgM ($\male$): 0.24–1.90 g/L
- IgM ($\female$): 0.75–2.30 g/L
- Electrophoresis: qualitative report given (e.g. monoclonal, polyclonal)

Background

- Immunoglobulins are proteins consisting of 2 heavy and 2 light chains produced by terminally differentiated B cells (or plasma cells) that are important in immunity
- There are 5 classes of immunoglobulin in normal serum, determined by their heavy chains: 80% is IgG, 15% IgA, 5% IgM, 0.2% IgD, with trace IgE
- Laboratory testing for immunoglobulins in blood typically detects IgG, A and M
- Immunoglobulin levels are age- and sex-dependent
- A small percentage of otherwise healthy individuals will statistically have immunoglobulin levels that fall just outside the reference ranges

Indication for testing

- Suspected immunodeficiency, e.g..
  - think Severe, Prolonged, Unusual or Recurrent (SPUR) infections without known cause
  - recurrent sinus/chest infection with *Strep. pneumoniae* or *H. influenzae*
  - failure to respond as expected to antimicrobial therapy
  - unexplained diarrhoea
  - FHx of immune deficiency
- Suspected monoclonal B-cell lymphoproliferative disease, e.g. myeloma, lymphoma or chronic lymphocytic leukaemia (CLL) (see *Chapter 2*)
  - immunoglobulins, protein electrophoresis and free light chain assessment (by checking urine Bence Jones proteins (BJP) or serum free light chains (sFLC)) should be tested to assess for paraprotein and associated suppression of normal immunoglobulins
  - serial monitoring can be used to assess disease progression, e.g. with monoclonal gammopathy of undetermined significance (MGUS)
- Assessing conditions with ↑ globulins, e.g.:
  - connective tissue disease
  - chronic liver disease
  - chronic infection: untreated HIV

Interpretation

- Depending upon the clinical condition, levels of the different antibody classes may be raised or reduced, or there may be a combined picture with ↑ in certain classes and ↓ in others
- Serum electrophoresis is required to determine whether an ↑ Ig level is monoclonal or polyclonal (there are different causes of both)
  - if a monoclonal Ig is identified, immunofixation is reflexed by the lab to type the monoclonal protein
  - serum Ig **must** be accompanied by serum electrophoresis and free light chain assessment (urine BJP or sFLC) to look for paraproteins
- Measurement of serum Ig does not provide categorical diagnosis of any disease
- Normal serum Ig do **not** exclude immunodeficiency, although in most cases, a normal full blood count (FBC) and Ig will be sufficient reassurance
- If no monoclonal protein is identified on serum electrophoresis and urine/serum free light chain assessment is normal, ↑ Ig is polyclonal

Causes of hypogammaglobulinaemia

- Primary (inherited)
  - can affect one or more Ig classes
  - rarer (apart from IgA deficiency)
- Secondary (acquired): more common
  - reduced Ig production:
    - malnutrition, alcoholism
    - medications, e.g. immunosuppressants, steroids, sodium valproate
    - malignancy, e.g. lymphoma
    - viral infection
  - increased Ig loss:
    - nephrotic syndrome, severe renal disease
    - protein-losing enteropathy

Causes of different patterns

Finding	Causes
↓ IgM	IgM levels ↓ with age: an isolated ↓ IgM, in the absence of a paraprotein, can be seen in adults >60 and is of doubtful clinical significance
	Medications
	Renal impairment
	Lymphoproliferative disease (rare)
↓ IgG	Loss from gut or kidneys

Finding	Causes
↓ IgA	Occurs in 1 in 200
	Commonly asymptomatic
	May have slightly ↑ risk of gastrointestinal diseases (including coeliac disease), autoimmune disease, or a modest increase in the rate of superficial infections
↓ 2 or more Ig classes	If features of immunodeficiency, consider referral to clinical immunologist

Causes of hypergammaglobulinaemia

- Monoclonal: output from one clonal B-cell population MGUS
  - seen in multiple myeloma or other B-cell lymphoproliferative disorders
  - causes ↑ in one Ig class (the paraprotein), which can be associated with suppression of the other two main classes
  - despite ↑ total Ig, patients can be immunocompromised as the abnormal protein does not contribute to protective immunity
  - causes:
    - MGUS
    - myeloma (IgG, IgA, less commonly IgM)
    - CLL
    - non-Hodgkin lymphoma
    - amyloidosis
    - Waldenström's macroglobulinaemia
- Polyclonal (reactive): output from multiple B-cell populations
  - seen with autoimmune or inflammatory disease and infection
  - multiple Ig classes are affected
  - causes:
    - liver disease: cirrhosis, chronic hepatitis
    - connective tissue disease: SLE, RA
    - acute and chronic infection: HIV, Epstein–Barr virus (EBV)
    - neoplasia
- Oligoclonal: output from a small number of B-cell populations
  - causes: chronic infection, autoimmunity and certain B-cell neoplasms

Causes of different patterns

Finding	Causes
↑ IgM	Non-specific marker of inflammation/infections
	Can be associated with PBC and sclerosing cholangitis
↑ IgG	CTD
	Sarcoid
	Liver disease
	HIV
	If clinically well no further Ix warranted

Finding	Causes
↑ IgA	Non-specific
	Common, especially in elderly
	Respiratory inflammatory disease
	GI inflammatory disease
	Liver disease
	Autoimmune conditions, e.g. RA, ankylosing spondylitis
	If clinically well no further Ix warranted
↑ 2 or more Ig classes	Chronic bacterial infection
	Sarcoid
	HIV

3.2.2 Total and specific IgE

Background

- Allergic disease is primarily a clinical diagnosis: tests are used to help confirm or refute a diagnosis
- Follow appropriate local testing and referral procedures

Total IgE

Normal range: 0–75 kU/L

- Indication for testing: measurement of total IgE is not indicated or essential in routine investigation of allergic disease
  - it should not be requested in isolation
  - specific IgE should always be requested with total IgE
- Interpretation:
  - ↑ in:
    - allergic disorders, e.g. atopic eczema, allergic asthma, allergic bronchopulmonary aspergillosis
    - parasitic diseases, e.g. invasive helminthiasis
    - autoimmune disease, e.g. pemphigoid, occasionally scleroderma
    - immunodeficiency conditions, e.g. hyper IgE syndrome

Specific IgE (formerly called RAST)

Normal range: results are expressed in terms of a grade or as a serum concentration of specific IgE, the units being kilounits of allergen-specific IgE per litre (kUA/L)
- Grade 0 = <0.35 kUA/L (negative)
- Grade 1 = 0.35–0.70 kUA/L (weak positive)
- Grade 2 = 0.7–3.5 kUA/L (positive)
- Grade 3 = 3.5–17.5 kUA/L (positive)
- Grade 4 = 17.5–52.5 kUA/L (strong positive)
- Grade 5 = 52.5–100.0 kUA/L (strong positive)
- Grade 6 = >100 kUA/L (strong positive)

- Indication for testing: specific IgE to suspected food, drug or inhalant triggers may be appropriate depending on the clinical circumstances – blanket testing is not helpful
  - specific IgE should always be requested with total IgE
  - do not test unless there is a typical history of immediate type allergy symptoms within an hour of contact with the allergen under investigation
  - these tests can be against single allergens, mixtures of related allergens (e.g. nut mix) or against mixtures of the most common allergens of one type (e.g. the inhaled allergen (aeroallergen) mix or the common food allergen mix)
  - IgE responses to more than 1000 allergens can be measured. Examples include:
    - rhinitis: cat dander and house dust mite
    - asthma and seasonal rhinitis pollens: grasses (May–September), trees (March–May) and weeds (July–September); months relate to the UK
    - asthma: house dust mite, animal dander (cats, dogs, horses)
- Interpretation:
  - allergy cannot be diagnosed on the basis of specific IgE tests alone
  - a positive specific IgE confirms sensitisation to the allergen tested: this may or may not be responsible for the cause of symptoms
  - a negative specific IgE does not exclude allergy, especially where there is a convincing history
  - a high total IgE can result in false positive specific IgE results: this is often found in those with atopic dermatitis, resulting in weakly positive results to multiple allergens due to non-specific IgE binding
  - false positive tests are common, e.g. wheat and hazelnut, due to cross-reactivity with grass and tree pollen allergy

3.3 Rheumatology

3.3.1 HLA-B27

Normal: negative

- Indication for testing: generally **not** a primary care investigation – check local protocols
  - NICE advises that this test can be considered in primary care if age <45 years and low back pain >3 months and 3 of the following are present, to help decide if rheumatology referral is needed (proceed with referral if positive):
    - low back pain starting before the age of 35
    - symptoms which wake them during the second half of the night
    - buttock pain
    - improvement when moving
    - improvement within 48 hours of taking a non-steroidal anti-inflammatory drug (NSAID)
    - spondyloarthritis in a 1st-degree relative
    - current or past arthritis
    - current or past enthesitis
    - current or past psoriasis

- Strongly associated with ankylosing spondylitis (present in 90% of patients), but not diagnostic
- Linked to other diseases, e.g. reactive arthritis, inflammatory bowel disease (IBD), uveitis
- Present in 8% of healthy individuals
- Not helpful as a screening test: only around 1% of positive individuals develop ankylosing spondylitis

3.3.2 Inflammatory markers: CRP/ESR/PV

Normal values:
C-reactive protein (CRP): <10 mg/L
Erythrocyte sedimentation rate (ESR): ♂ 0–22 mm/h; ♀ 0–29 mm/h
Plasma viscosity (PV): 1.50–1.72 mPa.s

Indication for testing

- Suspected infection or inflammatory disease
  - note these markers are non-specific
    - they ↑ in malignancy and infection
    - obesity causes ↑ CRP
    - ESR ↑ with age
    - PV is independent of age, sex, and Hb
- Monitoring disease activity and response to treatment, e.g. polymyalgia rheumatica (PMR)

Interpretation

- Check lab protocols for preferred inflammatory marker tests locally
- Normal inflammatory markers do not exclude rheumatological conditions: use clinical judgement and refer if concerns
- Testing multiple inflammatory markers does not improve the ability to rule out disease, but does increase the risk that at least one of the tests will give a false positive
- The overall diagnostic utility of all three inflammatory markers is similar and low
  - CRP marginally outperforms ESR and PV for infections (changes more rapidly)
  - CRP tends to be cheaper than ESR and PV
- Thus, CRP should generally be the 1st-line test, except in:
  - myeloma: ESR and PV are superior to CRP, but other relevant tests are needed if suspected (immunoglobulins, serum electrophoresis and free light chain assessment via urine BJP or sFLC)
  - suspected connective tissue disease: CRP can be normal, so ESR/PV are better
  - suspected giant cell arteritis (GCA): test CRP and either ESR or PV
  - suspected PMR: test CRP and either ESR or PV

What test should be used?

Scenario	CRP	ESR	PV	Comments
Acute infection	Y	N	N	CRP changes most rapidly
Suspected PMR?	Y	Y	Y	Test CRP and either ESR or PV
Suspected GCA?	Y	Y	Y	Test CRP and either ESR or PV
Suspected myeloma?	N	Y	Y	NICE advises ESR or PV
				If suspected, check the appropriate screen: serum electrophoresis and free light chain assessment (via urine BJP or sFLC)
Monitoring PMR?	Y	N	N	Useful when tapering steroids
				CRP is generally more sensitive
				No need to routinely test both CRP and ESR/PV
Suspected CTD?	N	Y	Y	CRP can be normal, so ESR/PV are better

3.3.3 Uric acid (urate)

Normal range: ♂ 200–430 µmol/L, ♀ 140–360 µmol/L

- Indication for testing:
  - suspected gout:
    - NICE advises to measure the serum urate level in acute suspected gout: a level of ≥360 µmol/L confirms the diagnosis in conjunction with appropriate signs and symptoms
    - gout should not be diagnosed on the presence of hyperuricaemia alone
    - if <360 µmol/L but gout is strongly suspected, check serum urate in 2–4 weeks after the flare has settled
  - titrating urate-lowering therapy for prevention
    - aim for a target serum urate level <360 µmol/L, but consider a lower target of <300 µmol/L for people with gout who:
      - have tophi or chronic gouty arthritis
      - continue to have ongoing frequent flares despite having a level <360 µmol/L
- May be ↑ in healthy individuals and by diuretics

References

References to support all aspects of testing and management guidance can be found, broken up by section, by scanning the QR code below or clicking on the Resources tab on the page for this book at www.scionpublishing.com/lab_results

Follow your local reference ranges, clinical pathways, management and referral guidance. This guidance is not a substitute for individual clinical judgement. Reference ranges will vary according to the assay used by laboratories. Those provided are examples and may vary in your locality.

4.1 Microscopy, culture and sensitivity (MCS) tests

4.1.1 Interpreting antibiotic sensitivity testing results

Background

- It is important to consider the clinical presentation and possible colonising flora present at different body sites (see table below)
- Consider if treatment is needed if the patient is asymptomatic: could this be colonising flora?
- Seek advice from a microbiologist if unsure of the significance of any results (not all scenarios are covered in the chapter)

Examples of normal flora in the body (not exhaustive)	
Site	**Example organisms**
Skin	*Candida* spp.
	Diphtheroids (*Corynebacterium*)
	Micrococcus
	Cutibacterium (previously known as *Propionibacterium*)
	Staphylococcus
	Streptococcus
Upper respiratory tract	May vary according to site, e.g. nose, pharynx
	• *Candida* spp.
	• *Staphylococcus*
	• *Streptococcus*
Gastrointestinal tract	Anaerobes, e.g. *Bacteroides*
	Lactobacillus spp.
	Enterococcus
	'Coliforms', e.g. many serotypes of *E. coli*, *Klebsiella* spp.
Female reproductive tract	*Candida* spp.
	Corynebacterium
	Enterococcus
	Lactobacillus spp.
	Staphylococcus
	Streptococcus
	Anaerobes

Urinary tract	Female urethra: • Anaerobes • *Corynebacterium* • *Lactobacillus* spp. • *Streptococcus* Male urethra: • *Corynebacterium* • *Streptococcus*
Oral cavity	*Staphylococcus* *Streptococcus* Anaerobes

Interpretation

Results are given in three susceptibility categories:

- **S** – 'Susceptible, standard dosing regimen': microorganism is thus categorised when there is a high likelihood of therapeutic success using a standard dosing regimen of the agent
- **I** – 'Susceptible, increased exposure*': microorganism is thus categorised when there is a high likelihood of therapeutic success because exposure to the agent is increased by giving it at a higher dose, increased frequency or at a higher concentration at the site of infection (by the fact that the agent concentrates naturally at the site of infection, e.g. many antibiotics become concentrated by secretion or filtration into the urine)
  - *exposure is a function of how the mode of administration, dose, dosing interval, infusion time, distribution and excretion of the antimicrobial agent will influence the infecting organism at the site of infection
  - seek advice in cases of renal impairment for optimal dosing regimen
- **R** – 'Resistant': microorganism is thus categorised when there is a high likelihood of therapeutic failure even when there is increased exposure

4.1.2 Nail clippings/scrapings MCS

Indications for testing

- Suspected fungal nail disease, if patient wishes to consider management with antifungal treatments, e.g. associated:
  - discomfort when walking
  - significant psychological distress due to the cosmetic appearance
  - comorbid conditions which increase the risk of complications, e.g. diabetes
  - fungal skin infection, with the nail infection being the likely source
- Advise that antifungal treatment is not needed if:
  - asymptomatic, and/or
  - not troubled by nail appearance (note that treatment may not successfully improve the appearance anyway)

Interpretation

- Interpret the results as positive if:
  - for dermatophytes, *either* microscopy or culture is positive
  - for *Candida* species, *both* microscopy and culture are positive
  - for non-dermatophytes, *both* microscopy and culture are positive on at least two samples taken at different times
- Testing for antifungal susceptibilities is not required
- Interpret the results with caution, as false-negative rates may be high (30%)
  - a negative test result cannot definitively exclude fungal nail infection
  - arrange repeat samples if the result is negative and there is a high clinical suspicion of fungal nail infection

GP management tips

- This depends on the site and severity of nail involvement, causative organism, symptoms and comorbidities
- Discuss patient expectations for successful management before starting treatment: onychomycosis is difficult to eradicate and often recurs
- Dermatophyte or *Candida* nail infection is confirmed:
  - option of topical antifungal treatment in adults if there is:
    - only very early, distal, and superficial nail involvement
    - superficial white onychomycosis
    - a contraindication to oral antifungal treatment
    - amorolfine 5% nail lacquer:
      - can be purchased over the counter
      - apply once or twice weekly to the affected nail(s) after gentle nail filing
      - treatment duration: 6 months for fingernails; 9–12 months for toenails
- Offer treatment with an oral antifungal agent if confirmed fungal nail infection and self-care measures and/or topical treatment are not successful or appropriate:
  - dermatophyte nail infection:
    - 1st-line: oral terbinafine 250 mg once a day
      - 6–12 weeks for fingernail infections
      - 12–24 weeks for toenail infections
    - 2nd-line: oral itraconazole pulsed therapy of 200 mg twice a day for 1 week, with subsequent courses repeated after a further 21 days
      - two pulses for fingernail infections
      - three pulses for toenail infections
  - *Candida* or non-dermatophyte nail infection:
    - 1st-line: oral itraconazole pulsed therapy of 200 mg twice a day for 1 week, with subsequent courses repeated after a further 21 days
      - two pulses for fingernail infections
      - three pulses for toenail infections
    - 2nd-line: oral terbinafine 250 mg once a day
      - 6–12 weeks for fingernail infections
      - 12–24 weeks for toenail infections

    o liver function test (LFT) monitoring is needed for terbinafine and itraconazole
- itraconazole:
  - monitor LFTs if treatment continues for >1 month, if receiving other hepatotoxic drugs, or if history of hepatotoxicity with other drugs
  - advise immediate LFTs if symptoms of possible liver toxicity develop, e.g. anorexia, nausea, vomiting, fatigue, abdominal pain or dark urine
- terbinafine:
  - should not be prescribed in people with chronic or active hepatic disease
  - hepatotoxicity may occur in people with and without pre-existing hepatic disease, therefore periodic monitoring of LFTs (after 4–6 weeks of treatment) is recommended
  - stop immediately if LFTs are deranged

4.1.3 Sputum MCS

Background

- Sputum samples are known to have issues with contamination: obtain early-morning samples as they contain pooled overnight secretions where pathogenic bacteria are more likely to be concentrated
- Collect the first sample before any antimicrobial therapy is initiated
- Note any current antibiotic therapy on the request form
- Fungal and TB cultures are not run as standard
- The most common pathogens detected are bacteria such as *Streptococcus pneumoniae, Haemophilus influenzae, Moraxella catarrhalis,* and *Klebsiella* species
- The presence of normal upper respiratory tract flora should be expected in sputum culture, e.g. *Neisseria* other than *N. meningitides* or *N. gonorrhoeae, Candida albicans,* diphtheroids, alpha-haemolytic streptococci, and some staphylococci

Indications for testing

- Chest infection
  - o use CRB-65 score to stratify mortality risk (the score is calculated by giving 1 point for each of the following prognostic features:
    - **C**: confusion (new disorientation in person, place or time; or abbreviated mental test score ≤8)
    - **R**: ↑ respiratory rate (≥30 breaths per minute)
    - **B**: ↓ blood pressure (systolic <90 mmHg or diastolic ≤60 mmHg)
    - **65**: age ≥65 years
      - score 0: low risk of death (<1% mortality risk)
      - score 1–2: intermediate risk (1–10% mortality risk)
      - score 3–4: high risk (>10% mortality risk)
  - o request a sputum culture for those with moderate-severity community-acquired pneumonia for whom community management is appropriate
  - o do not routinely recommend microbiological tests for people with low-severity community-acquired pneumonia

- Bronchiectasis
  o diagnosis is suspected: sputum microbiology is helpful in identifying the presence of persistent pathogens, especially *Pseudomonas aeruginosa*, which indicates a worse prognosis
    ▪ specialist follow-up is required for people with chronic colonisation with *P. aeruginosa*, opportunist *Mycobacteria,* or methicillin-resistant *Staphylococcus aureus* (MRSA)
  o acute exacerbations: prior to starting empirical therapy
- Chronic obstructive pulmonary disease (COPD)
  o diagnosis is suspected: only if sputum is persistently present and purulent
  o acute exacerbations: if managed in primary care, sputum cultures are not recommended in routine practice

Interpretation

- Culture results should be interpreted considering the signs and symptoms
- For all patients, consider antibiotic susceptibility results and resistance when deciding on initial management and/or reviewing antibiotic treatment if empirical treatment was started
- Note any comments included with culture results from the lab, e.g. 'likely colonising flora'
- Seek advice from a microbiologist if clinically needed or advised in the lab result

4.1.4 Stool MCS

Background

- Most cases of acute diarrhoea are mild and self-limiting
- No investigation or treatment is usually necessary, except in specific indications such as outbreaks, specific patient factors or relevant travel (see 'Indications for testing' below)
- Most laboratories will test all samples for *Salmonella, Shigella, Campylobacter, E. coli* O157, *Giardia* and *Cryptosporidium* as standard. This is often by polymerase chain reaction testing, as it is more sensitive than culture
- Document any relevant clinical history so that the lab reflexes tests for other relevant organisms, e.g. travel history, antibiotic use, shellfish consumption, farm visits
- Antibiotic susceptibility results are not usually reported, as treatment is not generally needed; in some cases (specifically Shiga toxin-producing *Escherichia coli* (STEC) – previously called verotoxigenic *E. coli* (VTEC)) it may make the illness worse
- Note that some infections and all cases of suspected food poisoning are notifiable by law to Public Health (Health Protection Team)

Indications for testing

- Symptoms/signs of infective diarrhoea, e.g.
  - systemically unwell
  - blood or pus in the stool
  - immunocompromised
  - recently received antibiotics, chemotherapy, on proton pump inhibitors (PPIs) or been in hospital (request specific testing for *Clostridioides difficile*)
  - foreign travel to anywhere other than western Europe, North America, Australia or New Zealand (request tests for ova, cysts and parasites and state the countries visited)
  - amoebiasis, giardiasis or cryptosporidiosis are suspected: if diarrhoea is persistent (≥2 weeks) or the person has travelled to an at-risk area
  - worsening symptoms in a patient with chronic bowel disease, e.g. irritable bowel syndrome (IBS), inflammatory bowel disease (IBD)
- Public health indication:
  - diarrhoea in high-risk people, e.g. food handlers, healthcare workers, elderly residents in care homes
  - suspected food poisoning, e.g. after a barbecue, restaurant meal or eating eggs/chicken/shellfish
  - outbreaks of diarrhoea in the family or community, when isolating the organism may help pinpoint the source of the outbreak
  - contacts of people infected with certain organisms where there may be serious clinical sequelae to an infection, e.g. *E. coli* O157 or *C. difficile*
  - close household contacts of a person with a giardia infection

Interpretation

- Usually only a single specimen is needed; repeat testing is unnecessary unless advised by a specialist (microbiologist or consultant in Public Health) or ova, cysts and parasites are suspected (send 3 specimens a minimum of 2 days apart)
- Most infective causes of diarrhoea do not require antibiotic treatment; seek advice from microbiologist if needed

GP management tips

Amoebiasis

- Seek specialist advice for confirmed cases: drug treatment is usually recommended, e.g. metronidazole followed by diloxanide
- Seek specialist advice regarding the need for microbiological clearance to confirm treatment success, 1 week after completing treatment

Campylobacteriosis

- Usually self-limiting; treatment is not usually needed for mild symptoms
- If severe symptoms (high fever, bloody and/or high-output diarrhoea) or immunocompromised, consider early prescribing with clarithromycin 250–500 mg twice daily for 5–7 days within 3 days of illness onset

Cryptosporidiosis

- Usually self-limiting; no specific treatment licensed in the UK
- Seek specialist advice if severely immunocompromised (risk of serious, life-threatening complications)
- Advise no swimming for 2 weeks after the last diarrhoea episode

E. coli

- Two types:
  - o STEC: Shiga toxin-producing *Escherichia coli* (STEC) – previously called verotoxigenic *E. coli* (VTEC)
  - o non-STEC
- STEC infection:
  - o there is no effective antibiotic treatment available for *E. coli* STEC infection: antibiotics are contraindicated as there is a theoretical risk of triggering haemolytic uraemic syndrome (HUS)
  - o seek specialist advice from Public Health on the need for stool testing for microbiological clearance in people at increased risk of transmission of infection, e.g. food handlers
    - ■ at least 2 consecutive negative stool samples are usually needed taken at least 24 hours apart, once the person is symptom-free for at least 48 hours, before the person can return to work or other institutional/social settings
  - o seek specialist advice regarding monitoring for the complication of HUS
- Non-STEC infection:
  - o seek specialist advice from Public Health regarding the need for exclusion and microbiological clearance in people at increased risk of transmission of infection, e.g. food handlers
    - ■ 2 consecutive negative stool samples are usually needed, the second sample taken 48 hours after the person is symptom-free, before the person can return to work, depending on a risk assessment

Giardiasis

- Prescribe metronidazole 2000 mg once daily for 3 days, or 400 mg three times daily for 5 days
- Advise no swimming for 2 weeks after the last episode of diarrhoea

Salmonellosis (non-typhoidal)

- Antibiotic treatment usually not needed
- Seek specialist advice on return to work, especially those who work with vulnerable groups, e.g. elderly and children, or food handlers

Shigellosis

- Mild symptoms: treatment usually not needed
- Severe symptoms (high fever, bloody and/or high-output diarrhoea) or immunocompromised: seek specialist advice on antibiotic treatment
- Advise on safe sexual practices if transmission amongst men who have sex with men (MSM) has resulted in an outbreak
- Seek specialist advice on the need for exclusion of cases from childcare or work settings, and the need for microbiological clearance stool testing (varies depending on the *Shigella* species)

Clostridioides difficile (formerly known as *Clostridium difficile*) infection (CDI)

Interpreting results:
- Labs undertake a two-stage testing approach which consists of:
  - stage 1: a test to detect the presence of *C. difficile*; depending on the lab, this may be glutamate dehydrogenase enzyme immunoassay (GDH EIA) or a nucleic acid amplification test (NAAT) or PCR
  - stage 2: a more specific EIA test for detecting toxin A&B produced by *C. difficile*
- If stage 1 is negative, the second test does **not** need to be performed
- If stage 1 and 2 are positive, CDI is likely to be present
- If stage 1 is positive and stage 2 negative, CDI could be present
- If stage 1 and stage 2 are negative, CDI could still be present; the type of test and patient symptoms need to be considered (NAAT and PCR are more specific, and therefore more predictive of CDI than GDH testing)

Management:
- Ideally seek prompt specialist advice before prescribing antibiotics, discussing:
  - any previous treatment for *C. difficile*
  - any concomitant antimicrobials
  - immunocompromise
  - severity of infection (admit if any severe/life-threatening signs)
    - **non-severe** – white cell count (WCC) <15 × 10^9/L, ≤50% ↑ in serum creatinine above the person's baseline level, and a core body temperature ≤38.5°C at presentation
    - **severe** – defined by one of the following features at presentation:
      - WCC ≥15 × 10^9/L
      - >50% ↑ in serum creatinine above the person's baseline level
      - core body temperature >38.5°C

- **fulminant** (previously known as life-threatening or severe-complicated) – defined by any of the following features attributed to CDI:
  – hypotension
  – evidence of septic shock
  – evidence of ileus, toxic megacolon or bowel perforation
  – rapid deterioration in clinical condition
- General treatment principles:
  o review whether PPIs and H$_2$ antagonists can be substituted with simple antacids, e.g. alginates, while antibiotic therapy is required
  o discontinue laxatives
  o review medications which may cause problems if people are dehydrated, e.g. NSAIDs, ACE inhibitors (ACEi), angiotensin receptor blockers (ARBs), diuretics
  o avoid anti-motility agents, e.g. loperamide
  o avoid drugs with anti-peristaltic effects, e.g. opioids
  o review currently prescribed antimicrobials and discontinue unless necessary
  o if oral (or via established enteral feeding tube) medication cannot be taken, consider admission
- If awaiting a *C. difficile* test result and it is highly suspicious that the person has CDI, assess the severity and consider seeking specialist advice on whether empirical antibiotic treatment should be offered
- If CDI is confirmed, consider seeking prompt specialist advice (from microbiologist or infectious disease specialist) before prescribing antibiotics
- Antibiotic treatment:
  o first episode of non-severe CDI: vancomycin 125 mg orally 4 times a day for 10 days
  o 2nd-line antibiotic for a first episode of non-severe CDI: fidaxomicin 200 mg orally twice a day for 10 days
  o 1st- and 2nd-line antibiotics are ineffective: seek specialist advice
  o further episode of CDI within 12 weeks of symptoms resolution (relapse): fidaxomicin 200 mg orally twice a day for 10 days
  o further episode of CDI after 12 weeks of symptoms resolution (recurrence): vancomycin 125 mg orally 4 times a day for 10 days *or* fidaxomicin 200 mg orally twice a day for 10 days
- Follow-up:
  o routine clearance samples should not be sent
  o samples from previously positive patients will not routinely be retested within 28 days
  o clearance samples may still be positive due to colonisation with *C. difficile*, which does not require treatment if the patient is well and asymptomatic
  o repeat samples are only necessary if the patient is clinically unwell or symptomatic
  o use clinical judgement to determine whether antibiotic treatment is ineffective
    - it is not usually possible to determine this until day 7, as diarrhoea may take 1–2 weeks to resolve

- if the person's condition has improved considerably or has resolved without treatment, consider the possibility of a false-positive test result
- if antibiotics have been started and subsequent stool sample tests do not confirm CDI, consider stopping these antibiotics

4.1.5 Urine MCS

Background

- Due to high throughput, most diagnostic laboratories will use an automated machine to process 'microscopy' requests
- Depending on the clinical details and microscopic results, the urine may then be cultured and incubated overnight
- All urines that are considered negative by microscopy will not receive a culture and the result will be authorised immediately (except in special indications)
- Paediatric urine testing is not covered in this section

Indications for testing: dipstick or MCS?

- For suspected urinary tract infection (UTI) in adults, dipstick testing is not recommended for all groups
- Definitions:
  - uncomplicated UTI: caused by typical pathogens, in non-pregnant women, with no known urinary tract abnormalities and no predisposing comorbidities
  - complicated UTI: have an increased likelihood of complications, e.g. treatment failure, persistent/recurrent infection, in those with risk factors, e.g. pregnant women, urinary tract abnormalities, indwelling urinary catheters, renal disease, immunocompromised

Interpretation

- Culture should be interpreted considering signs and symptoms: false negatives or positives can occur
- Do not treat asymptomatic bacteriuria, unless pregnant
- Follow-up samples are not usually indicated, except when treating asymptomatic bacteriuria in pregnancy

Urine testing: when to dipstick vs. send for MCS

Group	Dipstick or MCS?	Notes
Pregnant	Send urine MCS	Arrange repeat urine MCS once antibiotic treatment is completed, to ensure clearance of infection
Concerning symptoms	Send urine MCS	These include: • Suspected sepsis/pyelonephritis (send urine MCS for sample collected before antibiotics are taken, but do not delay treatment) • Has symptoms that are persistent, not resolving with antibiotic treatment, or recurring within 4 weeks after antibiotic treatment • Has visible or non-visible haematuria • Recurrent UTI (2 episodes in last 6 months, or 3 episodes in last 12 months) • Atypical symptoms
Risk factors for antibiotic resistance or complicated UTI	Send urine MCS	Risk factors for complicated UTI: • Pregnancy • Post-menopause • 'Healthcare-associated' UTI (in long-term care or hospital settings) • Virulent or atypical infecting organisms and multi-drug-resistant organisms • Recent urologic instrumentation, e.g. catheterisation • Pre-existing urological conditions, e.g. childhood UTI and vesicoureteral reflux; recurrent UTIs; neurogenic bladder due to multiple sclerosis or spinal cord injury; polycystic kidney disease; renal transplant; renal stone disease; and urinary tract structural abnormality • Comorbidities, e.g. diabetes mellitus, immunocompromised Risk factors for antibiotic resistance: • Structural abnormality of the genitourinary tract • Renal impairment • Being in long-term care • Being hospitalised for more than 7 days in the last 6 months • Recent travel to a country with increased antibiotic resistance • Previous resistant UTI • Prolonged use of antibiotics • Recurrent UTI

Group	Dipstick or MCS?	Notes
Catheter-associated UTI	Send urine MCS	Do **not** use urine dipsticks: most adults with a catheter *in situ* for >1 month will have asymptomatic bacteriuria and results will most likely be unhelpful Arrange for an indwelling urinary catheter to be ideally removed (or replaced) before starting antibiotic treatment, if possible • If the catheter has been changed, the sample should be collected from a newly placed catheter (using an aseptic technique, drain a few ml of residual urine from the tubing, then collect a fresh sample from the catheter sampling port). Do *not* collect the sample from the urine collection bag • If the catheter has been removed, obtain a mid-stream urine (MSU) sample

Women age <65 with suspected uncomplicated UTI	>1 key symptom present (dysuria, new nocturia, urine cloudy):
	• No dipstick or MCS needed
	
	1 key symptom present **or** any other urinary symptoms (frequency, suprapubic tenderness, urgency, visible haematuria):
	• Check dipstick
		UTI likely; treat as per guidance
		
		Sample containers with boric acid preservative should not be used to perform urine dipstick testing, as it can affect results
		
		Dipstick interpretation:
		• **Positive** nitrite or both **positive** leucocyte and RBCs **positive**:
		  ○ UTI likely
		• **Negative** nitrite and **positive** leucocyte with RBCs **negative**:
		  ○ UTI equally likely to other diagnosis
		  ○ send urine MCS to narrow differential, continue to consider other diagnoses
		• **Negative** for all nitrite, leucocyte and RBC:
		  ○ UTI less likely
		  ○ suggests an alternative cause for symptoms
		  ○ do not send urine MCS

Group	Dipstick or MCS?	Notes

		• If only **positive** for red blood cells (RBC): consider further referral for urgent suspected cancer assessment according to NICE guidelines
		  ○ haematuria (visible and unexplained) either without UTI or that persists or recurs after successful treatment of UTI, age ≥45 (bladder or renal cancer)
		  ○ haematuria (non-visible and unexplained) with dysuria or raised WCC on a blood test, age ≥60 (bladder cancer)
		  ○ haematuria (visible) with low haemoglobin levels or thrombocytosis or high blood glucose levels or unexplained vaginal discharge in women age ≥55 (endometrial cancer, consider direct access USS pelvis)

Men age <65	Send urine MCS	• Collect urine MCS before antibiotics are given
		• Dipsticks are unreliable at ruling out infection; however, they may be helpful in some clinical situations to decide if a working diagnosis of UTI should be made:
		  ○ a dipstick with **positive** nitrites makes UTI more likely in men (PPV 96%)
		  ○ a dipstick **negative** for nitrites and leucocytes makes UTI less likely, especially if symptoms are mild

Adult men or women aged >65 with suspected uncomplicated UTI	Assess the symptoms, and send urine MCS if:
	• New onset dysuria alone, or
	• 2 or more of:
	  ○ temperature 1.5°C above patient's normal twice in the last 12 hours
	  ○ new frequency or urgency
	  ○ new incontinence
	  ○ new or worsening delirium / functional decline
	  ○ new suprapubic pain
	  ○ visible haematuria
		Do **not** use urine dipsticks: there are high rates of bacteriuria in this age group which do not need treating

Growth counts

- Many labs use growth of 10^7–10^8 cfu/L (10^4–10^5 cfu/ml) to indicate UTI
- Lower counts can also indicate UTI if the patient is symptomatic:
  - strongly symptomatic women: single isolate >10^5 cfu/L (>10^2 cfu/ml)
  - men: counts as low as 10^6 cfu/L (10^3 cfu/ml) of a pure or predominant organism
  - any single organism >10^7 cfu/L (>10^4 cfu/ml)
  - *Escherichia coli* or *Staphylococcus saprophyticus* >10^6 cfu/L (>10^3 cfu/ml)
  - >10^8 cfu/L (>10^5 cfu/ml) of a predominant organism (even with small amounts of mixed growth)
  - group B Streptococci (GBS) in pregnant women: intrapartum antibiotic prophylaxis should be offered to women with GBS bacteriuria identified during the current pregnancy; those with GBS urinary tract infection (growth >10^5 cfu/ml) should receive appropriate treatment at the time of diagnosis as well

Epithelial cells / mixed growth

- The presence of epithelial cells is not necessarily an indicator of perineal contamination: interpret with symptoms and repeat if of uncertain significance
- Mixed growth may indicate perineal contamination, but a small proportion of UTIs may be due to genuine mixed infection; consider re-test if symptomatic

Red cells

- May be present in UTI
- Lab microscopy for red cells is less accurate than dipstick due to red cell lysis in transport
- Refer patients with persistent haematuria post-UTI to urology

White blood cells / leucocytes

- White cells >10^7 WBC/L (>10^4 WBC/ml) are considered to represent inflammation in the urinary tract, including the urethra
- White cells can be present in older people with asymptomatic bacteriuria, as the immune system does not differentiate colonisation from infection

Sterile pyuria

- Consider *Chlamydia trachomatis* (especially if age 16–24 years), other sexually transmitted diseases, vaginal infections, other non-culturable organisms (including TB), or renal pathology
- False negative cultures may arise if the patient is taking antibiotics prior to producing a urine sample
- If recurrent pyuria with UTI symptoms, discuss with local microbiologist, as lower counts down to 10^5 cfu/L (10^2 cfu/ml) may be significant. Higher volumes of urine may need to be cultured, including for fastidious organisms

Antibiotic susceptibility

- For all patients, consider antibiotic susceptibility results and resistance when deciding on management and for reviewing antibiotic treatment if empirical treatment was started

- Refer to relevant NICE antimicrobial guidance, e.g.
  - UTI (lower): antimicrobial prescribing (NG 109)
  - pyelonephritis (acute): antimicrobial prescribing (NG 111)
  - catheter-associated UTI: antimicrobial prescribing (NG 113)

4.1.6 Vaginal discharge MCS

Background

- Vaginal discharge may be:
  - physiological: white or clear, mucus-like, non-offensive discharge that varies with the menstrual cycle and in the different reproductive stages
  - pathological: change in colour, consistency, volume and/or odour; may be associated with symptoms such as itch, soreness, dysuria, pelvic pain, or intermenstrual or post-coital bleeding
- Abnormal vaginal discharge can be due to:
  - infective (non-sexually transmitted) causes, e.g. bacterial vaginosis (BV), candidiasis
  - infective (sexually transmitted) causes, e.g. chlamydia, gonorrhoea
  - non-infective causes, e.g. retained foreign body, dermatitis, cancer
- Check the appropriate sample has been taken for the suspected infection and write clinical details on the request
- High vaginal and cervical swabs: black-topped charcoal swabs should be used for routine sampling, e.g. thrush, BV
- Specific swabs are available for *Chlamydia* and *N. gonorrhoeae* detection from the cervix, urethra and limited other sites
- *Chlamydia* and *N. gonorrhoeae* can be detected in urine samples, but this test is not available in all labs, and will require a specific transport medium

Indications for testing

- High vaginal swabs may be used to aid diagnosis of BV, vulvovaginal candidiasis, *Trichomonas vaginalis*, or other genital tract infections, such as streptococcal organisms; their use should generally be reserved for when:
  - symptoms, signs or pH are inconsistent with a specific diagnosis
  - the woman is pregnant, postpartum, post-abortion, post-miscarriage, post-instrumentation, or pre-or post-gynaecological surgery
  - it is within 3 weeks of intrauterine contraceptive insertion
  - symptoms are recurrent (≥4 cases a year)
  - there is no, partial, or poor response to treatment
- Those at increased risk of a sexually transmitted infection (STI) (e.g. those who have condomless sex with new or casual partners, *or* are <25 years of age, *or* have had a new sexual partner or more than one sexual partner in the last 12 months, *or* have had a previous STI, *or* are of Black ethnicity) should be offered testing for chlamydia, gonorrhoea, trichomoniasis, HIV and syphilis
  - ideally, testing should be done in a genitourinary medicine (GUM) clinic to facilitate treatment and partner notification

   o   if unwilling or unable to attend a GUM clinic, testing can be done in primary care

Interpretation

- Manage isolates as per local protocols and guidance
- Seek specialist advice in paediatric, pregnant and breastfeeding patients

GP management tips

Bacterial vaginosis (not pregnant)

- Asymptomatic: treatment is not usually required, other than in the context of having some gynaecological procedures
- Symptomatic: oral metronidazole 400 mg twice a day for 5–7 days
  - o   if adherence is an issue, a single oral dose of 2 g may be used
  - o   if topical treatment preferred or cannot tolerate oral metronidazole: intravaginal metronidazole gel 0.75% once a day for 5 days (off-label for women aged <18 years) or intravaginal clindamycin cream 2% once a day for 7 days

Chlamydia (not pregnant)

- If suspected or confirmed, strongly recommend referral to a GUM clinic for management
  - o   if the person declines, or is unable to attend a GUM clinic, manage uncomplicated genital chlamydia infection in primary care
- First-line: doxycycline 100 mg twice daily for 7 days (contraindicated in pregnancy and breastfeeding)
- If doxycycline is contraindicated or not tolerated, consider azithromycin 1 g orally as a single dose for 1 day, followed by 500 mg orally once daily for 2 days
- If doxycycline or azithromycin are contraindicated, consider erythromycin 500 mg twice daily for 10–14 days
  - o   ofloxacin 200 mg twice daily for 7 days, or 400 mg once daily for 7 days is a possible alternative (beware MHRA warnings for quinolone use)

Gonorrhoea

- All patients should be referred to a GUM clinic or other local specialist sexual health service. If the person is unwilling or unable to attend this, primary care management can be undertaken if the appropriate expertise is available and in line with local procedures and protocols

Trichomoniasis

- Ideally, treatment should be provided by a GUM clinic or other local specialist sexual health service. If this is declined or not possible, the person should be managed in primary care
- Women (not pregnant or breastfeeding):
  - o   prescribe oral metronidazole 400–500 mg twice a day for 5–7 days, or metronidazole 2 g as a single oral dose
  - o   seek advice from a GUM specialist if the person has a confirmed metronidazole allergy

Vulvovaginal candidiasis (not pregnant)

- Advise on antifungal drug treatment options and preparations, depending on the woman's age, comorbidities, personal preference, and drug cautions and contraindications
- 1st-line:
  - fluconazole 150 mg oral capsule as a single dose 1st-line, *or*
  - clotrimazole 500 mg intravaginal pessary as a single dose if oral therapy is contraindicated
- Vulval symptoms: add clotrimazole 1% or 2% cream applied 2–3 times a day
- Severe:
  - fluconazole 150 mg oral capsule on days 1 and 4 1st-line, *or*
  - miconazole nitrate 1.2 g single-dose vaginal capsule: insert 1 capsule intravaginally once at night on days 1 and 4
- Alternative regimens (if 1st-line oral azole or intravaginal imidazole therapy is contraindicated or not tolerated for acute infection):
  - intravaginal creams
    - clotrimazole 10% cream: 5 g intravaginally, single dose at night
    - miconazole 2% cream: 5 g intravaginally once at night for 7 nights
  - intravaginal pessaries
    - clotrimazole 200 mg pessaries (3 pessaries): insert 1 pessary intravaginally once at night for 3 nights
    - econazole nitrate 150 mg single-dose pessary: insert 1 pessary intravaginally once at night as a single dose
    - econazole nitrate 150 mg pessaries (3 pessaries): insert 1 pessary intravaginally once at night for 3 nights
    - miconazole nitrate 1.2 g single-dose vaginal capsules: insert 1 capsule intravaginally once at night as a single dose
    - miconazole nitrate 400 mg vaginal capsule: insert 1 capsule intravaginally once at night for 3 nights
    - fenticonazole 200 mg vaginal capsules (3 capsules): insert 1 capsule intravaginally once at night for 3 nights
    - fenticonazole 600 mg single-dose vaginal capsules: insert 1 pessary intravaginally once at night as a single dose
  - oral itraconazole: 200 mg twice a day for 1 day
  - severe infection
    - clotrimazole 500 mg pessary (2 pessaries): insert 1 pessary intravaginally on days 1 and 4
    - miconazole nitrate 1.2 g single-dose vaginal capsule: insert 1 capsule intravaginally once at night on days 1 and 4

Group B Streptococcus (GBS) (not pregnant)

- A vaginal commensal in 10–15% of women
- No evidence that GBS in isolation increases the risk of pelvic inflammatory disease (PID)
- Asymptomatic carriers do not require treatment
- Consider treatment advice if post termination, or gynaecological surgery
- Pregnant women will need assessment for intra-partum prophylaxis

4.2 Specific testing

4.2.1 Cervical screening and human papillomavirus (HPV)

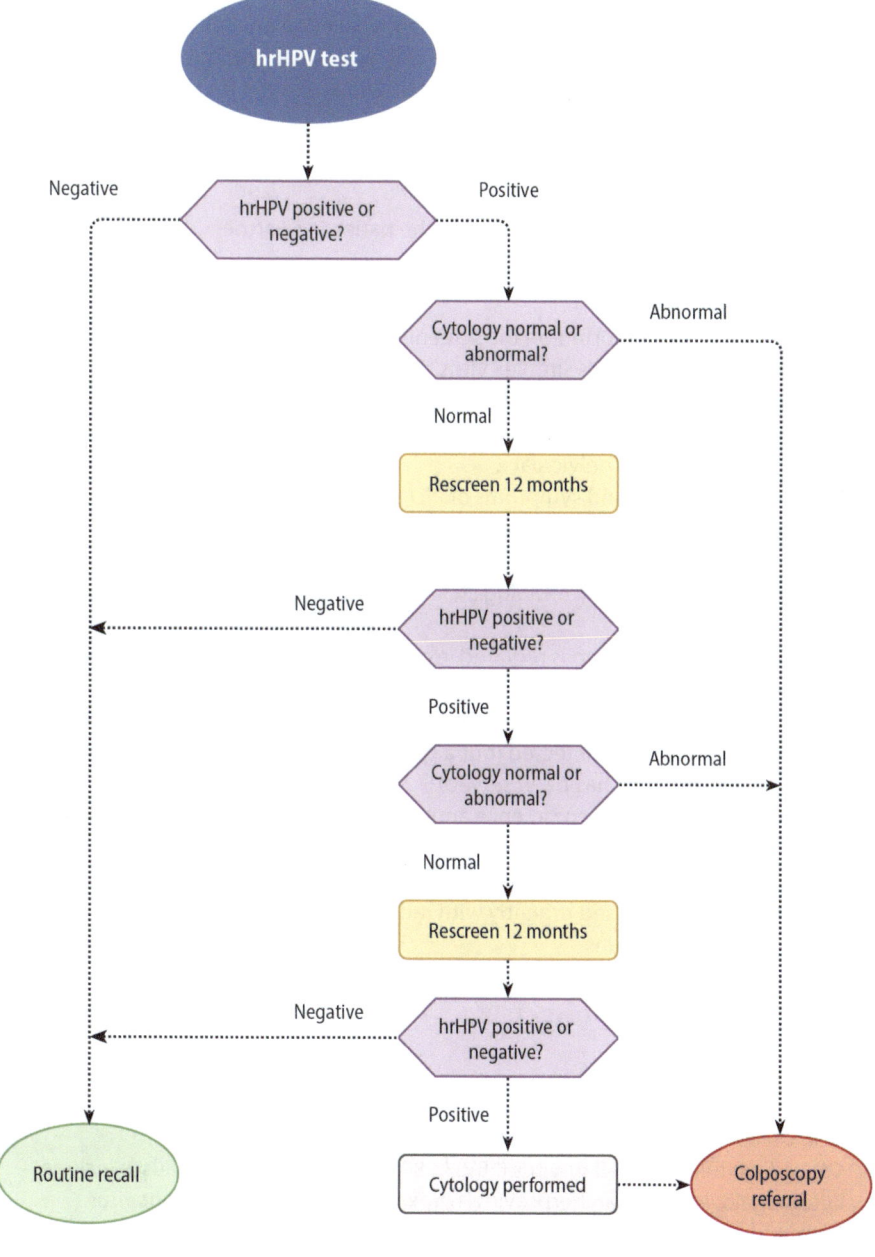

Background

- Cervical screening in the UK involves:
  - primary human papillomavirus (HPV) screening: to identify people with high-risk HPV (hrHPV)
  - liquid-based cytology: if hrHPV is found
  - colposcopy: to diagnose cervical intraepithelial neoplasia (CIN) and differentiate high- and low-grade lesions in people with abnormal cytology
- Women are invited at different ages and intervals across the four nations in the UK

Interpretation

- The actions and recall are automated
- HPV does not need specific treatment in the patient or partner

GP management tips

- Manage organisms reported on the screening report as per guidelines, e.g. *Candida*, bacterial vaginosis, herpes simplex virus, *Trichomonas vaginalis*
- If actinomyces-like organisms (ALOs) are present on cervical screen report, manage as follows:
  - if symptomatic, e.g. pelvic pain:
    - assess for signs and symptoms of PID
    - assess for other more common causes of pain, including STIs
    - if intrauterine contraception is *in situ*, consider removing it
    - seek advice from microbiologist
  - if asymptomatic:
    - no specific follow-up is required, e.g. in terms of the need for repeat swabs for ALOs
    - there is no immediate need to remove intrauterine contraception just because ALOs are detected (but a coil should never remain *in situ* indefinitely once its purpose has been served)
    - there is no need to commence antibiotic treatment: this is likely colonisation vs. infection
    - if ever actinomycosis is suspected, further investigation and management should be discussed urgently with radiology, microbiology and/or gynaecology teams

4.2.2 Glandular fever

Background

- Also called infectious mononucleosis
- Caused by the Epstein–Barr virus (EBV) in 80–90% of cases; other causes include cytomegalovirus, human herpesvirus 6, toxoplasmosis, HIV and adenovirus
- Commonest between 15 and 24 years old

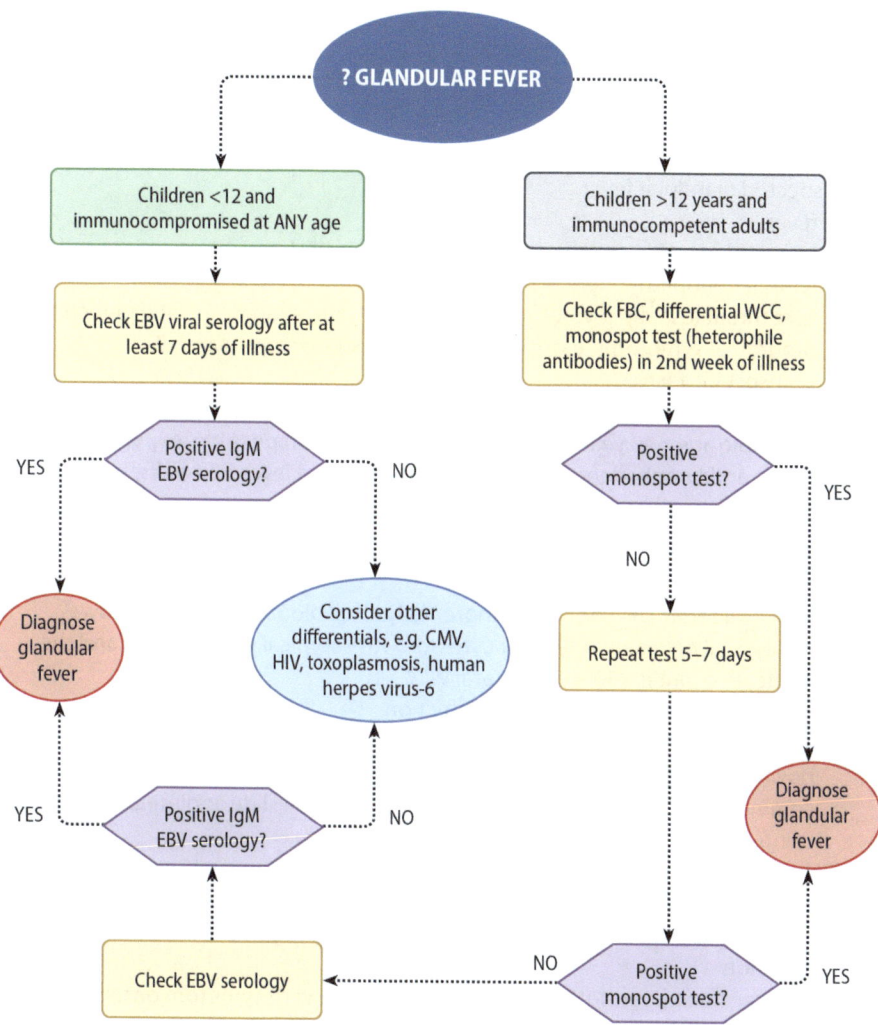

- Spread mainly through contact with saliva, but can be via semen and blood
- Incubation period: 4–7 weeks
- Complications:
  - hepatitis
  - upper airways obstruction
  - cardiac, e.g. pericarditis, myocarditis
  - renal, e.g. interstitial nephritis
  - neurological, e.g. encephalitis, aseptic meningitis, facial nerve palsy, MS
  - haematological, e.g. mild thrombocytopenia (25–50%), autoimmune haemolytic anaemia (3%), splenic rupture (<1%)

- o chronic fatigue (10%)
- o cancer, e.g. Hodgkin's lymphoma
- Prognosis: self-limiting in most, lasting 2–4 weeks. EBV remains in the body lifelong

Indications for testing

- Suspected glandular fever
  - o fever
  - o lymphadenopathy: mildly tender, mobile, typically bilateral posterior cervical lymphadenopathy
  - o sore throat (usually severe): tonsillar enlargement, exudate, palatal petechiae
  - o prodromal symptoms, e.g. general malaise, fatigue, myalgia, chills
  - o non-specific rash
  - o hepatosplenomegaly
  - o in people age >40 years: more atypical presentation possible, e.g. without sore throat and lymphadenopathy (>50%), unexplained fever >2 weeks, jaundice (20%)

Interpretation

- FBC, WCC differential: diagnosis is more likely if full blood count (FBC) shows >20% atypical or 'reactive' lymphocytes, or >10% atypical lymphocytes and the lymphocyte count is >50% of the total WCC
- Monospot test: non-specific for EBV infection
  - o IgM antibodies agglutinate red cells from other species (sheep, horse, goat, bovine)
  - o commonly used monospot test is a rapid qualitative slide agglutination test using horse or bovine red cells
- EBV antibodies: in patients with symptoms and lymphocytosis, but negative heterophile antibodies, testing for EBV-specific antibodies is indicated
  - o the specific antigens are important for distinguishing between acute and past infection
  - o viral capsid antigen-IgM (VCA-IgM) is detectable with symptom onset in most, peaking at 2–3 weeks and is then unmeasurable by 4 months
  - o VCA-IgG peaks at 2 to 3 months and persists for life
  - o EBV nuclear antigen (EBNA) antibodies rise in resolution phase and remain detectable for life. These develop after 6–8 weeks and can be used to identify past infection, or as evidence to rule out acute EBV infection

GP management tips

- Most only require supportive measures at home
- Avoid heavy lifting and contact/collision sports for the first month of the illness, to reduce the risk of splenic rupture
- Consider LFTs: transaminase elevations are usually transient and mild (2–3× the upper limit of normal)

4.2.3 Helicobacter pylori (H. pylori)

Background

- *H. pylori* infection is one of the most common causes of peptic ulcer disease
- NSAID use may have an additive effect if there is co-existent *H. pylori* infection
- Also associated with acute and chronic gastritis, gastric cancer and gastric mucosa-associated lymphoid tissue (MALT) lymphoma
- Its presence should be confirmed before starting eradication treatment
- Consider local protocols for initial testing and retesting:
  - recommended initial tests can be either of these three (check local pathways):
    - urea (13C) breath test
      - should not be performed within 2 weeks of PPI use or 4 weeks of antibacterial treatment, as this can lead to false negatives
      - most accurate test
      - needs a prescription and staff time to perform
    - stool antigen test (SAT)
      - should not be performed within 2 weeks of PPI use or 4 weeks of antibacterial treatment, as this can lead to false negatives
      - pea-sized piece of stool sent to local laboratory
    - laboratory-based serology (where locally validated)
      - lower accuracy
      - not recommended for most patients: positives should be confirmed by a second test, e.g. urea breath test or SAT or biopsy
      - detects IgG antibody: does not differentiate active from past infection, so not appropriate to use after treatment
  - for re-testing:
    - use urea (13C) breath test
    - perform at least 4 weeks (ideally 8 weeks) after treatment
    - if requiring gastric acid suppression, H_2-receptor antagonists should be used

Indications for testing

Initial testing may be undertaken in the following:
- Uncomplicated dyspepsia and no alarm symptoms who are unresponsive to lifestyle changes and antacids, following a single one-month PPI treatment course
- High risk of *H. pylori* infection, e.g. older people, north African ethnicity (test first or in parallel with PPI course)
- Previously untested with a history of peptic ulcers or bleeds
- Prior to initiating NSAIDs in patients with a prior history of peptic ulcers or bleeds
- Unexplained iron-deficiency anaemia after endoscopic investigation has excluded malignancy, and other causes have been investigated

Retesting is recommended as follows:
- Poor compliance
- High local resistance rates

- Persistent symptoms and the initial test was performed within 2 weeks of PPI treatment or within 4 weeks of antibacterial treatment
- Associated peptic ulcer, MALT lymphoma or after resection of early gastric carcinoma
- Taking aspirin without concomitant PPI
- Severe persistent or recurrent symptoms, particularly if not typical of gastro-oesophageal reflux disease

Interpretation

- Positive *H. pylori* testing warrants eradication therapy (triple-therapy)
- Triple-therapy regimen: comprises a PPI and two antibacterials
- Choice of antibacterials should take into consideration the patient's antibacterial treatment history: each additional course of clarithromycin, metronidazole or quinolone increases the risk of resistance
- Do not use clarithromycin or metronidazole if used in the past year for any infection
- Recommended PPI doses: lansoprazole 30 mg, omeprazole 20–40 mg, esomeprazole 20 mg, pantoprazole 40 mg or rabeprazole 20 mg
- If diarrhoea develops while on or up to 1 month after antibiotic therapy, consider test for *C. difficile* infection

H. pylori eradication therapy guide: no penicillin allergy				
Treatment	PPI e.g.	Antibiotic 1	Antibiotic 2	Duration
1st-line	Omeprazole 20 mg BD or lansoprazole 30 mg BD	Amoxicillin 1 g BD	Clarithromycin 500 mg BD or metronidazole 400 mg BD	7 days
2nd-line	Omeprazole 20 mg BD or lansoprazole 30 mg BD	Amoxicillin 1 g BD	Whichever was not used 1st-line Clarithromycin 500 mg BD or metronidazole 400 mg BD	7 days
Alternative 2nd-line (previous clarithromycin and metronidazole in the last 1 year)	Omeprazole 20 mg BD or lansoprazole 30 mg BD	Amoxicillin 1 g BD	Levofloxacin 250 mg BD or tetracycline hydrochloride 500 mg QDS	7 days

- Consider referral to a specialist if remains *H. pylori*-positive after 2nd-line eradication therapy
- Patients should be referred for an endoscopy, culture and susceptibility testing if the choice of antibacterial treatment is reduced due to hypersensitivity, there are known high local resistance rates, or patients have previously received treatment with clarithromycin, metronidazole and a quinolone

H. pylori eradication therapy guide: penicillin allergy					
Treatment	**PPI e.g.**	**Antibiotic 1**	**Antibiotic 2**	**AND**	**Duration**
1st-line	Omeprazole 20 mg BD or lansoprazole 30 mg BD	Clarithromycin 500 mg BD	Metronidazole 400 mg BD	–	7 days
Previous use clarithromycin	Omeprazole 20 mg BD or lansoprazole 30 mg BD	Metronidazole 400 mg BD	Tetracycline hydrochloride 500 mg QDS	Bismuth subsalicylate 525 mg QDS	7 days
2nd-line, no previous exposure to levofloxacin	Omeprazole 20 mg BD or lansoprazole 30 mg BD	Metronidazole 400 mg BD	Levofloxacin 250 mg BD	–	7 days
2nd-line, previous exposure to levofloxacin	Omeprazole 20 mg BD or lansoprazole 30 mg BD	Metronidazole 400 mg BD	Tetracycline hydrochloride 500 mg QDS	Bismuth subsalicylate 525 mg QDS	7 days

4.2.4 Hepatitis B

Background

- Diagnosis of hepatitis B virus (HBV) is based on the presence of serological markers (antigens and antibodies) in plasma or serum
- Provide full clinical details to allow selection of the appropriate tests, including:
  - vaccination status
  - if the test is for past exposure or response to vaccination

- o if acute hepatitis is suspected
- o if immunocompromised (in some cases, testing HBV-DNA may be more useful)
- Requests for hepatitis B serology lead to a panel of tests which may differ from lab to lab: use clinical judgement to determine the range of required tests, depending on the suspected diagnosis, and seek specialist advice if unsure
  - o initial testing should ideally include (at least) HBsAg and anti-HBc
  - o further tests may be required depending on the findings, e.g. hepatitis B e antigen, or antibody status (anti-HBe), HBV DNA level, IgM antibody to hepatitis B core antigen (anti-HBc IgM)
  - o positive HBsAg and positive anti-HBc IgM confirm an acute infection, particularly if supported by clinical suspicion and raised ALT
  - o positive HBsAg and anti-HBc (total or IgG) but negative anti-HBc IgM confirm a chronic infection
  - o different combinations of antibodies and antigens, alongside other findings, can indicate the phase of a chronic infection, which is used in determining appropriate treatment options

Indication for testing

- Asymptomatic people who are at high risk of hepatitis B infection, e.g.
  - o born or brought up in a country with intermediate or high prevalence
  - o current or historic injecting drug users
  - o change sexual partners frequently
  - o sex workers
  - o close contacts of a person with HBV infection
  - o families adopting children from countries with a high or intermediate prevalence of hepatitis B, and foster carers
  - o receiving haemodialysis for chronic kidney disease (CKD)
  - o chronic liver disease
  - o living in supported living accommodation, including residential care for those with learning disabilities
  - o history of sexual assault
  - o sustained a needlestick injury, other sharps injury or bite
- People with clinical features suggestive of hepatitis B infection:
  - o acute infection:
    - a prodromal illness that includes fever, arthralgia or a rash (that may appear about 2 weeks before the onset of jaundice, then resolves)
    - non-specific malaise (which may be profound), fatigue, nausea and poor appetite
    - right upper quadrant abdominal pain
    - jaundice (with dark urine and/or pale stools if cholestasis is present)
    - extrahepatic manifestations, e.g. glomerulonephritis, vasculitis and polyarteritis
  - o chronic infection:
    - often no physical signs or symptoms
    - possible signs of chronic liver disease after many years of infection,

depending on the severity and duration, e.g. spider naevi, finger clubbing, jaundice, palmar erythema, hepatosplenomegaly; in severe cases: thin skin, bruising, ascites, liver flap and encephalopathy
- People with abnormal LFTs:
  - acute hepatitis B:
    - ALT and AST may ↑ significantly (usually 500–10 000 IU/L)
    - bilirubin may be ↑ (can reach up to 500 µmol/L)
    - ALP is usually < twice the upper limit of normal, but can be higher in the presence of cholestasis
    - PT may be prolonged (≥5 seconds suggests severe hepatitis and ≥50 seconds suggests acute liver failure)
  - chronic hepatitis B:
    - for most, the only indicator is a mildly ↑ serum aminotransferase level; in many, liver enzymes will be normal

Interpretation

The following may be tested and reported:
- **Hepatitis B surface antigen (HBsAg):**
  - indicates presence of viral envelope
  - suggests that the person is infectious
  - rises during the incubation period and may be cleared early in the course of the disease
  - undetectable in around 10% of people by the time the test is performed
  - chronic HBV infection is indicated by the persistence of serum HBsAg for >6 months
- **Hepatitis B e antigen (HBeAg):**
  - detectable in the serum during both the early phases of acute infection and some chronic infections
  - usually associated with relatively high levels of virus replication
  - people with chronic HBV tend to be more infectious if HBeAg is detected
  - if HBeAg has been cleared, anti-HBe is usually detected, and infectivity is lower
- **Antibody to HBeAg (anti-HBe):**
  - present following clearance of HBeAg from the plasma
  - disappearance of HBeAg, development of anti-HBe, and a decline in HBV-DNA indicates control of viral replication and predicts resolution of acute hepatitis B
- **Antibody to HBcAg (anti-HBc):**
  - indicates current or previous HBV infection
  - appears at the onset of symptoms in acute infection and generally persists for life
  - may be absent very early in acute infection
- **IgM antibody to hepatitis core antigen (anti-HBc IgM)**
  - indicates recent (within the last 6 months) HBV infection
  - quantification may be useful to distinguish between acute and chronic infection
  - usually replaced gradually by IgG anti-HBc
- **IgG antibody to hepatitis core antigen (anti-HBc IgG):**

- o generally persists for life and is indicative of past infection
- **Antibody to HBsAg (anti-HBs):**
  - o indicates recovery from and immunity to HBV
  - o anti-HBs without anti-HBc is a marker of immunisation
  - o anti-HBs is quantified to measure vaccination response
- **Quantification of HBV DNA (HBV viral load)**
  - o high levels of HBV DNA are associated with a greater risk of progression to cirrhosis and hepatocellular cancer
- **HBV core avidity testing**
  - o can differentiate between acute and chronic core IgM infection

Guide to interpretation of hepatitis B serology tests (variations do occur and the local lab will normally provide a result interpretation)

Test Scenario	HBsAg	Anti-HBs	HBeAg	Anti-HBe	Anti-HBc (IgG)	Anti-HBc (IgM)	HBV DNA	ALT
Acute hep B infection	+	−	+	−	+	+	+	↑
Immunity following infection	−	+	−	+/−	+	−	−	Normal
Immunity from vaccination	−	+	−	−	−	−	−	Normal
Susceptible (consider vaccination)	−	−	−	−	−	−	−	Normal
Chronic hep B: active	+	−	+/−	+/−	+	−	+	↑
Chronic hep B: inactive carrier	+	−	−	+	+	−	+ (low)	Normal

4.2.5 Hepatitis C

Background

- Hepatitis C virus (HCV) infection is diagnosed with:
  - o an antibody test: this indicates if a person has ever been infected with HCV
  - o HCV RNA test by PCR: checks if infection is active and for genotype analysis
- In immunocompetent people, send a sample for testing for antibodies to HCV
- If the antibody test is positive, or in immunocompromised people, send a blood sample for HCV RNA

- If a healthcare professional has, or may have, sustained an occupational exposure to HCV, e.g. from a needlestick injury:
  - advise that they will need HCV antibody testing at 12 and 24 weeks, and HCV RNA testing at 6, 12 and 24 weeks via their Occupational Health department

Indication for testing

- Offer screening to asymptomatic people who are at high risk of HCV infection, e.g.
  - history of injecting drugs
  - received a blood transfusion before 1991 or blood products before 1986, when screening of blood donors for hepatitis C infection, or heat treatment for inactivation of viruses, were introduced
  - born or brought up in a region/country with an intermediate or high prevalence (≥2%) of chronic hepatitis C, including Africa, Asia, the Caribbean, Central and South America, eastern and southern Europe, the Middle East, and the Pacific islands
  - babies born to mothers infected with hepatitis C
  - prisoners, including young offenders
  - looked-after children and young people, including those living in care homes
  - living in hostels for the homeless or sleeping on the streets
  - HIV-positive MSM
  - close contacts of someone known to be chronically infected with hepatitis C, including family members, close friends, household contacts or sexual partners
- Consider testing people who are at increased risk of HCV infection, particularly if they have non-specific or unexplained symptoms and signs:
  - this includes the following groups:
    - history of snorting or smoking drugs (such as cocaine), particularly if they have shared straws or pipes
    - at risk through sharing of contaminated items, e.g. razors or toothbrushes
    - healthcare workers who have been accidentally exposed to blood where there is a risk of hepatitis C, e.g. needlestick injuries
    - received medical, cosmetic or dental treatment (or any other invasive treatment) in countries where hepatitis C is common and infection control may be poor (including people who have received blood transfusion products that have not been screened for hepatitis C)
    - had tattoos, body piercing, acupuncture or electrolysis, where unsterilised equipment may have been used (especially consider tattooing and piercing received in the UK before the mid-1980s or in other countries at any time)
    - tested positive for hepatitis B or HIV: HIV-positive MSM should be offered regular testing for hepatitis C
  - clinical features may include:
    - non-specific fatigue, myalgia, anxiety, depression, poor memory or concentration (may be indicative of chronic hepatitis C infection)
    - nausea and vomiting
    - right upper quadrant abdominal pain

- jaundice (with dark urine and/or pale stools if cholestasis)
- signs of chronic liver disease (in advanced chronic hepatitis C)
- Consider testing people with abnormal LFTs

Interpretation

- Antibodies to HCV:
  - positive (indicates resolved or current HCV infection):
    - test a second blood sample to confirm the diagnosis
    - consider taking an additional blood sample at the same time as the first sample if venepuncture is difficult, e.g. injects drugs
  - negative:
    - consider repeating it (especially if the person is at high risk of infection) at the appropriate time if the last risk exposure occurred within the 3–6-month 'window period' of the test
      - it can take at least 3 months for antibodies to become detectable: seek specialist advice if there is uncertainty about the optimal time to repeat the test
- HCV RNA PCR:
  - positive:
    - this means the person has current infection with active hepatitis C
    - send a repeat sample for confirmation
    - refer to specialist clinic for antiviral treatment
  - negative:
    - repeat the test after a period of 6 months
      - if the negative result is confirmed, this means the person has a previously resolved HCV infection, but they are not immune to future HCV infection
- If the person has equivocal results, or there is uncertainty interpreting the results, seek specialist advice
- If the person tests negative for HCV but remains at increased risk of infection, offer annual testing

4.2.6 HIV

Background

- There are two methods for routine testing:
  - laboratory-based tests performed on samples obtained through venepuncture
  - self-sampling, self-testing and rapid point-of-care tests (POCTs) which can be performed in the clinic, in the community setting or as a home test
- Consensus guidelines recommend 4th-generation HIV laboratory tests with venous sampling as the 1st-line choice, with POCTs also available (which are largely 3rd-generation tests)
- Note the 'window period': this is the time between becoming infected and antibodies appearing. HIV antibodies usually appear 4–6 weeks after infection, but can take up to 12 weeks

- Knowledge of window periods guides clinicians to offer the appropriate test, at the most appropriate time, and to advise patients accordingly. Factors governing the window period include characteristics of the virus, the test and the exposed individual's immune response
- HIV tests have evolved considerably, yielding progressive reduction in window periods over time; if unsure, check with local lab and repeat using a 12-week window
- The following window periods are applied when utilising the following tests:
  - 4th-generation lab tests: 45 days
  - 3rd-generation lab tests: 60 days
  - all POCTs (including Determine HIV-1/2 Ab (3rd generation), INSTI HIV-1/2 test and the OraQuick Rapid HIV-1/2 antibody test): 90 days
- Confirmatory testing should be undertaken according to locally determined pathways in liaison with local virology teams

Indications for testing

- Offer an HIV test in primary care (or where appropriate, direct to specialist services) to people who:
  - request testing
  - have risk factors for HIV, e.g.
    - have a current or former partner who is infected with HIV
    - from an area with high HIV prevalence
    - MSM
    - female sexual contacts of MSM
    - trans women
    - had multiple sexual partners, engage in high-risk sexual practices such as 'chemsex', or have a history of other STIs, e.g. syphilis, chlamydia
    - history of injecting drug use
    - current or previous sex workers
    - rape victims
    - had blood transfusions, transplants or other risk-prone procedures in countries without rigorous procedures for HIV screening
    - had an occupational exposure, e.g. needlestick injury
  - have another STI
  - have an AIDS-defining condition, an indicator condition, or clinical features of HIV infection
  - are newly registered with general practice or are having a blood test, if they have not had an HIV test in the past 12 months, in areas of the UK where diagnosed prevalence of HIV is high (>2 per 1000 population aged 15–59 years); annually updated HIV prevalence data by locality is available from the Public Health England website
  - are pregnant, as part of routine antenatal care

Interpretation

- Positive test
  - indicates HIV infection
  - result likely to be phoned through and a repeat sample advised
  - it does not indicate date of infection
  - refer patient to specialist HIV clinic
- Negative test
  - consider if a further test is needed to cover the window period
  - post-exposure prophylaxis, pre-exposure prophylaxis (PrEP) and early anti-retroviral therapy (ART) initiation in acute infection can blunt the HIV antibody response yielding non-reactive, atypical or non-progressive HIV serology in a setting in which the HIV viral load is likely to be undetectable; refer for specialist review

4.2.7 Lyme disease

Background

- Lyme disease is an infection caused by a specific group of bacteria, *Borrelia burgdorferi*, transmitted to humans following a bite from an infected tick
- Can result in several clinical problems ranging from skin rash to serious involvement of organ systems, including arthritis, and neurological problems
- Make a clinical diagnosis of Lyme disease in people with erythema migrans; no laboratory testing is required
- For people without erythema migrans, clinical presentation and laboratory testing is used to guide diagnosis and treatment
- Do not rule out the diagnosis if tests are negative but there is high clinical suspicion
- Consider starting treatment while awaiting test results

Indications for testing

- Suspected Lyme disease (but if erythema migrans is present, then start antibiotics without further testing)
- Serological testing is a two-tier approach: a sensitive initial test is performed first (ELISA), followed by a more specific confirmatory test (immunoblot) in case of a positive or equivocal initial result

Interpretation

- The chart below outlines the indications and appropriate timelines for lab tests:
- Healthcare professionals wishing to discuss a case or find out about local provision for testing for Lyme disease should contact their local consultant in microbiology or infectious diseases
- Immunoblot test: this should not be offered without discussion with a specialist
- People with erythema migrans and no focal symptoms (e.g. neurological, cardiac or joint involvement) should be prescribed oral antibiotics:

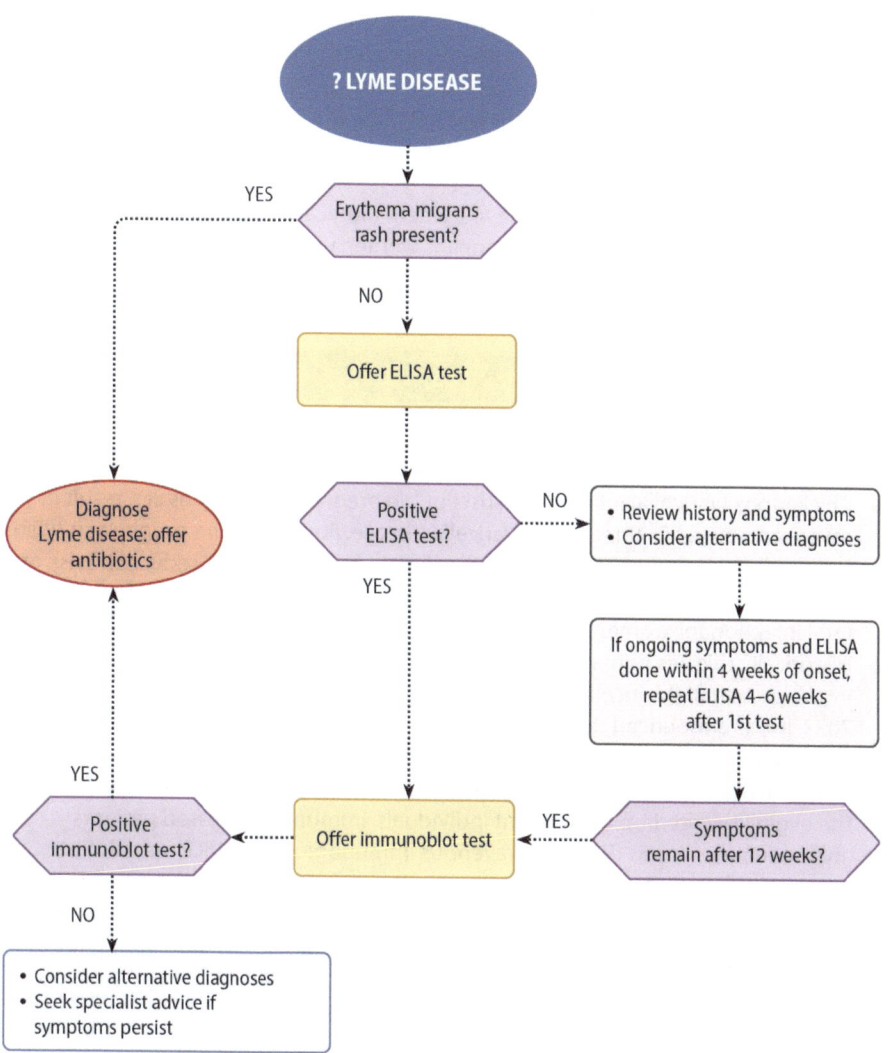

- o doxycycline 100 mg twice daily (or 200 mg once daily) for 21 days, *or*
- o amoxicillin 1000 mg three times daily for 21 days, *or*
- o azithromycin 500 mg daily for 17 days
- People with focal symptoms should be referred to the appropriate specialist, but treatment should not be delayed

4.2.8 Pregnancy and viral serology

- This section discusses the management of exposure to suspected varicella zoster virus, measles, parvovirus B19 and rubella in pregnant individuals; these are the most common types of viral rash illness encountered in the UK

- Management will vary according to whether the person has symptoms or not; seek urgent advice from the appropriate specialists for those with clinical signs/symptoms of disease
- Note that other rash illnesses, e.g. mpox and Zika virus, may also cause significant fetal problems, but are not discussed further here: follow local pathways if suspected
  - these are usually suspected due to epidemiological links or lifestyle factors
  - guidance suggests testing all pregnant women with a rash illness for syphilis; note most UK cases of congenital syphilis are due to maternal acquisition *after* the 12 weeks 'booking bloods'

Chickenpox (varicella zoster virus, VZV)

Background

- Chickenpox (varicella) infection in susceptible pregnant individuals can result in severe and even life-threatening varicella disease. Post-exposure prophylaxis (PEP) is recommended to reduce the severity of maternal disease and reduce the risk of complications, e.g. pneumonitis, in addition to a theoretical reduction in the risk of fetal infection for women contracting varicella in the first 20 weeks of pregnancy
- Historically this has primarily been achieved through the timely administration of intramuscular (IM) varicella zoster immunoglobulin (VZIG) in those at risk, but in 2023, it was announced that IM VZIG would no longer be produced by the supplier, and that current stock expired 30 September 2024
- Thus antivirals are now recommended for PEP for all at-risk groups who meet the eligibility criteria, e.g. pregnant individuals, immunosuppressed patients and neonates; a bolus dose of intravenous immunoglobulin (IVIG) may also be considered for eligible groups for whom oral antivirals are contraindicated
- PEP is recommended for individuals who fulfil all three of the following criteria:
  - significant exposure to chickenpox (varicella) or shingles (zoster) during the infectious period
  - susceptible pregnant women (at any stage of pregnancy)
  - no antibodies to VZV
- For all people with a history of exposure to chickenpox, establish whether the:
  - diagnosis of chickenpox in the contact is certain
  - exposure was significant enough to put the person at risk of infection
  - person has had chickenpox in the past
- Significant exposure considers the:
  - type of varicella zoster infection in the index case. Exposure is significant if the person has had contact with:
    - chickenpox
    - disseminated zoster
    - immunocompetent people with exposed lesions, e.g. ophthalmic zoster
    - immunocompromised people with localised zoster on any part of the body (this group may have increased viral shedding)

- timing of exposure in relation to the rash onset in the index case. Exposure is significant if the person was in contact with:
  - chickenpox: from 24 hours before onset of rash to crusting of lesions
  - disseminated zoster: from 48 hours before onset of rash to crusting of lesions
  - localised zoster: day of onset of rash until crusting of lesions
- closeness and duration of contact. Exposure is significant if it is through:
  - maternal/neonatal contact
  - continuous exposure, e.g. household member, nursery or care worker
  - >1 exposure to a case of chickenpox or shingles, e.g. family friend who visited on more than one occasion during the infectious period
  - contact in the same room, e.g. house or classroom for 15 minutes or more, or contact on large open wards (particularly paediatric wards)
  - face-to-face contact, e.g. having a conversation
- Perform a general assessment to establish the woman's risk of chickenpox, based on her history of chickenpox, the certainty of chickenpox in the contact, and the level of exposure

Indication for test

- VZV serology: presence confirms evidence of immunity from past infection or immunisation
- If a pregnant woman has a definite history of chickenpox or shingles or two doses of a varicella-containing vaccine, and is not immunocompromised, there is no risk of chickenpox and no need for serology testing (reassure the patient that immunity can be assumed)
- If a pregnant woman has no history of chickenpox or shingles (or is uncertain) and has a history of significant contact, establish the stage of gestation and seek urgent specialist advice
  - VZV IgG testing can help identify who would benefit from VZ PEP. This can be undertaken on booking bloods samples; liaise with the lab
  - note that PEP can be given from day 7–14 after the first day of exposure, allowing adequate time for bloods to be assessed

Interpretation

- Positive VZV IgG earlier than 48 hours following exposure (i.e. before any antibody response has had time to occur following current exposure) is evidence of immunity from past infection or immunisation
  - reassure she is immune
- Negative antibody status:
  - antiviral PEP is recommended if VZV IgG is <100 mIU/ml
  - oral aciclovir or valaciclovir is now the first choice PEP for all susceptible pregnant women at any stage of pregnancy
  - oral aciclovir or valaciclovir should be given from day 7 to day 14 after the first day of exposure. The day of exposure is defined as the date of onset of rash if the

index is a household contact and date of first or only contact if the exposure is on multiple or single occasions, respectively

- o aciclovir: 800 mg 4 times a day for 7 days, start course on day 7 after exposure; if the patient presents after this, the course may be started up to day 14 after exposure
- o valaciclovir: 1000 mg 3 times a day for 7 days, start course on day 7 after exposure; if the patient presents after this, the course may be started up to day 14 after exposure
- o in individuals where oral antivirals are contraindicated, IVIG may be considered, e.g. due to malabsorption or renal toxicity: arrange via local pathways, e.g. Obstetrics/Gynaecology service
- o women who have a second exposure during pregnancy should be risk assessed and if there was no evidence of symptomatic infection, have a repeat VZV antibody test on a fresh blood sample
- o further doses of PEP following second exposure: if there is a second or subsequent exposure to chickenpox or shingles within the first 7 days of PEP treatment, the course of antivirals may need to be extended until 14 days after the first day of exposure. If the exposure occurs ≥8 days after the first exposure, then a new course of antivirals should be started at day 7 following the second exposure, assuming repeat antibody testing for IgG is still negative – if repeat testing for IgG is positive, i.e. seroconversion has occurred, then obstetrics / fetal medicine advice should be sought

GP management tips

- Advise all women to promptly seek advice if they develop a rash and/or symptoms and have had contact with chickenpox (regardless of whether they have received antivirals or IVIG, or have a history of chickenpox, shingles or varicella vaccine
- For a pregnant woman with rash and chickenpox/shingles contact history:
  - o seek immediate obstetric advice regarding further management, e.g. antiviral treatment for the mother (note dose and duration differ from those for PEP) and outpatient follow-up for the fetus/newborn
  - o assess the need for hospital admission, e.g. respiratory or neurological symptoms, haemorrhagic rash or bleeding, severe disease (dense rash with or without mucosal lesions), significant immunosuppression (including recent use of systemic corticosteroids)

Measles

Background

- Complications of measles can be more severe in pregnant women, including miscarriage, premature birth, intrauterine death and stillbirth, and maternal death; there is no evidence of associated congenital defects
- Measles is a notifiable disease

- Suspected measles, pregnant women:
  - immediately notify the local Health Protection Team (HPT), who will advise on public health measures, including contact tracing to identify vulnerable individuals, and arrange surveillance testing
  - seek immediate obstetric advice
- Asymptomatic, pregnant women, possible measles contact:
  - determine the person's immunisation status, whether they are immunocompromised and whether they have had significant contact with a suspected case of measles
  - immediately notify the local HPT

Indication for test

- Pregnant women with suspected measles infection or asymptomatic with possible measles exposure
- Follow the guidance of the local HPT on testing; they will also know whether the presumed infectious contact definitely has measles
- In the UK, oral fluid (OF) is the optimal sample for measles diagnosis; this is minimally invasive and can be tested for IgM, IgG and measles RNA
  - OF cannot be used to assess the immune status of vulnerable contacts; serum should be used instead
  - IgM antibodies are positive in >50% of samples on day 1 of the rash, and in over 90% by day 3 of the rash
  - the relative level of measles IgG can be used to predict whether the case is a primary or breakthrough infection with measles
  - measles viral RNA can be detected from before the onset of the rash and for at least 2 weeks after the onset of symptoms
- In the absence of an OF sample, serum and a mouth swab should tested
- Serum samples:
  - can be used for IgM/IgG detection through enzyme immunoassays
  - are generally not suitable for PCR detection and viral typing
  - cannot distinguish wild-type measles from vaccine-derived measles following recent vaccination
  - may still be IgM negative within 3 days of onset of rash
  - serum can be used to confirm breakthrough measles (reinfection) by detection of high-avidity measles IgG
- Mouth swabs:
  - can be used for PCR if collected within 6 days of the onset of rash, but a negative PCR result does not exclude a diagnosis of measles
  - can distinguish between wild-type virus and vaccine in someone who has recently been vaccinated
  - cannot be used for measles IgM/G testing and cannot be used to distinguish between a primary infection and a breakthrough measles (reinfection)

Interpretation

Measles IgM and IgG interpretation

Test	IgM	IgG	Interpretation
Results	+	–	Active measles infection, as IgM antibodies are produced early in the infection phase
	–	+	Past measles infection or vaccination, as IgG antibodies persist long-term after exposure
	+	+	May indicate a recent infection where the immune system is still producing both types of antibodies
	–	–	No prior exposure to measles virus and lack of immunity

- Management of pregnant contacts
  - the aim of measles PEP for pregnant women is attenuation of disease: human normal immunoglobulin (HNIG) can be used
  - this will be issued up to 6 days after exposure, allowing time for assessment of immunity status in most instances
  - HNIG is not effective in reducing severity once infection/rash has developed
  - where a second exposure occurs >3 weeks after a first dose of immunoglobulin, a further dose may need to be considered
  - pregnant women who remain susceptible should be reminded to have measles, mumps and rubella (MMR) vaccination following delivery, to protect them in subsequent pregnancies
  - recommendations for pregnant women are based upon a combination of age, history and/or antibody testing:

Managing pregnant contacts of measles

Birth year	History of infection or vaccine	Action
Born before 1990	History of measles infection	Assume immune
	No history of measles infection	Test measles IgG
		Administer HNIG within 6 days only if measles antibody negative
	History of 2 measles-containing vaccines	Assume immune
Born 1990 or later	History of 2 measles vaccines	Assume immune
	History of 1 measles vaccine	Test measles IgG
		Administer HNIG within 6 days only if measles antibody negative
	Unvaccinated	Test measles IgG
		Administer HNIG if measles antibody negative
		If not possible to test within 6 days of exposure, offer HNIG

GP management tips

- Suspected measles, pregnant women:
  - give advice to:
    - stay away from nursery, school or work for at least 4 days after the initial development of the rash (ideally until full recovery to reduce the risk of infective complications)
    - avoid contact with susceptible people, e.g. not fully immunised by vaccination or natural exposure, infants, pregnant women or immunosuppressed
    - seek urgent medical advice if they develop complication, e.g. shortness of breath, uncontrolled fever
- Asymptomatic, pregnant women, possible measles contact:
  - seek advice about risk assessment for PEP

Parvovirus B19

Background

- Maternal infection can result in:
  - non-immune hydrops fetalis: occurs in 3–11% of cases if infection occurs between 9 and 20 weeks' gestation, and may cause fetal loss in about 40–50% of cases, if untreated
  - fetal death (5–10%)
- There is no vaccine or PEP available
- Relevant history:
  - symptomatic
    - pregnancy gestation
    - onset date, clinical features, rash type and distribution
    - previous relevant history of infection, antibody testing and vaccines received for other rash illnesses (with dates/places)
    - recent travel history and relevant dates
    - known contact with any person with a rash illness, or recent travel (with dates and destination(s) of travel and contact dates)
  - asymptomatic, possible parvovirus B19 exposure
    - assess if any significant contact and when with any person with a potentially infectious rash or illness (including before the onset of rash)
      - significant contact is defined as being in the same room for 15 minutes or more, or face-to-face contact with the person
      - household (rather than occupational) exposure is the most important source of infection in pregnancy
    - pregnancy gestation
    - previous history of infection, IgG antibody testing, and measles/rubella vaccination status (with dates/places)

- In suspected infection or asymptomatic exposure, contact the local virology, microbiology or infectious diseases department immediately for further advice on what lab tests and monitoring should be arranged. This should include:
  - confirming the diagnosis of parvovirus B19 infection
  - checking for rubella infection at the same time, irrespective of previous testing or immunisation status to rubella

Indication for test

- Symptomatic and asymptomatic pregnant women with possible parvovirus B19 exposure
- Parvovirus serology: IgM and IgG may be tested

Interpretation

- Symptomatic pregnant women: likely to have urgent blood testing for:
  - parvovirus B19-specific IgM: this can confirm or exclude infection by blood tests taken from the day after rash onset. Booking bloods or earlier samples may be available to aid diagnosis, but initial blood tests should not be delayed
    - not detected:
      - excludes infection in the 4 weeks prior to the blood test
      - infection cannot be excluded if the blood test is taken more than 4 weeks after the rash illness onset
    - detected in the first 20 weeks of pregnancy:
      - suggests recent infection with parvovirus B19
      - refer urgently to fetal medicine
      - confirmation is recommended by an alternative assay, e.g. high levels of B19V DNA or IgG seroconversion using booking blood
  - other rash illnesses, e.g. rubella, irrespective of previous testing or immunisation status to rubella
- Asymptomatic pregnant women with possible parvovirus B19 exposure: likely to have urgent blood testing for:
  - parvovirus B19-specific IgG and IgM (see table)
  - other rash illnesses, e.g. rubella, irrespective of previous testing or immunisation status to rubella

Parvovirus IgM and IgG interpretation			
Test	**IgM**	**IgG**	**Interpretation**
Results	–	+	Reassure
			Shows past (but not recent) infection
			Confirms immunity
			Retesting is not necessary
			Seek medical advice if symptoms of rash illness develop
	–	–	Indicates susceptibility to infection
			Repeat blood test 1 month after last contact, even if she remains asymptomatic (or earlier if symptoms develop)

			Interpreting bloods after 1 month:
			• Negative for both IgG and IgM:
			  ○ reassure there is no evidence of recent infection
			  ○ she remains susceptible to future infection
			• Positive for IgM and negative for IgG: urgent referral to fetal medicine and repeat blood test immediately to confirm results as suggests recent infection
			  ○ if remains positive for IgM:
			    ■ suggests recent infection
			    ■ confirmation is recommended by an alternative assay, e.g. high levels of B19V DNA or IgG seroconversion using booking blood

	+	+ or –	Suggests recent infection
			Urgent referral to fetal medicine and seek urgent specialist advice on any additional testing needed
			Diagnosis is confirmed by testing an antenatal booking blood sample or a repeat blood test after 7–10 days (to assess changes in IgM reactivity)

GP management tips

- Symptomatic
  - **urgent referral to fetal medicine for monitoring and management**
  - admit if acute complications, e.g. suspected severe anaemia
  - it is not usually necessary to stay off work if symptoms are controlled, as the infection is no longer contagious by the time the rash or arthropathy develops
  - if the woman has not been fully immunised against rubella or does not have a documented history of previous rubella infection, it may be sensible to avoid contact with other pregnant women while any rash is present, until her rubella status is known

- Asymptomatic
  - advise to avoid contact with other pregnant women and people at risk of complications, until she is known to be uninfected, immune to infection, or no longer potentially infectious; the infectious period can be up to 10 days before onset of rash, including the day of onset

Rubella

Background

- Rubella is generally a mild infection, but it can cause serious complications in pregnancy (congenital rubella syndrome; CRS). The risk of serious congenital defects is highest in the first trimester of pregnancy
- There are no effective treatments to prevent CRS; HNIG is not recommended routinely for PEP in pregnant women as there is no evidence that it is effective, but it may be considered in secondary care when termination of pregnancy is unacceptable
- Suspected rubella in pregnant women:
  - contact the local HPT immediately
    - rubella is a notifiable disease
    - testing for other infections with similar clinical features (e.g. parvovirus B19 and measles) may be carried out simultaneously
    - laboratory investigation is necessary for all pregnant women regardless of previous testing, immunisation status, or stage of pregnancy; they will advise on appropriate investigations
- Asymptomatic, pregnant women with possible rubella exposure:
  - contact the local HPT immediately
    - the status of the index case can be reviewed
    - investigations for other infections with similar clinical features (e.g. parvovirus B19 and measles) may be necessary
  - assess if she fulfils the criteria for immunity: evidence of protection against rubella includes at least two documented doses of rubella vaccine, or at least one rubella antibody screening test (before or at the time of exposure) that detected IgG antibodies:
    - yes, fulfils immunity criteria: reassure her that the likelihood of rubella infection is remote, that no investigation for rubella is necessary, but she must return if a rash develops
    - no, does not fulfil immunity criteria: arrange serology testing as soon as possible, stating the patient is pregnant

Indication for test

- Pregnant women with suspected rubella infection or asymptomatic with possible rubella exposure who do not meet the criteria for immunity
- Rubella serology: IgM and IgG may be tested

Interpretation

Rubella IgM and IgG interpretation			
Test	IgM	IgG	Interpretation
Results	–	+	Reassure that shows evidence of protection against rubella
			Advise her to return if a rash develops
	–	–	The woman is susceptible to rubella
			Retest after 4 weeks
	+	+ or –	Confirms rubella infection
			Arrange a second confirmatory test • First 20 weeks gestation (or any doubt about gestational age): urgent referral fetal medicine for CRS assessment • Gestation is confirmed >20 weeks: reassure no reported cases of CRS after this gestational age, referral to fetal medicine for management advice

GP management tips

- Suspected or confirmed rubella in pregnant women:
  - advise all women to:
    - stay off work for at least 5 days after the initial rash development (may be infectious up to 10 days post-rash)
    - avoid contact with other pregnant women
    - inform clinical staff prior to attending medical areas until known to be non-infectious or uninfected
    - seek urgent medical advice if symptoms do not improve or complications develop
- Asymptomatic, pregnant women with possible rubella exposure:
  - advise the woman to inform their midwife, GP or obstetrician urgently if they develop a rash at any time in pregnancy. Until they are assessed and confirmed to be uninfected or non-infective, they should:
    - avoid contact with other pregnant women
    - inform clinical staff of suspected infection prior to attending any medical area
  - arrange follow-up for unvaccinated women to be immunised with MMR vaccine after delivery: rubella immunisation should *not* be administered in pregnancy

4.3 List of notifiable diseases

- Acute encephalitis
- Acute infectious hepatitis
- Acute meningitis
- Acute poliomyelitis
- Anthrax
- Botulism
- Brucellosis
- Cholera
- Covid-19
- Diphtheria
- Enteric fever (typhoid or paratyphoid fever)
- Food poisoning
- Haemolytic uraemic syndrome (HUS)
- Infectious bloody diarrhoea
- Invasive group A streptococcal disease
- Legionnaires' disease
- Leprosy
- Malaria
- Measles
- Meningococcal septicaemia
- Mpox (previously known as monkeypox)
- Mumps
- Plague
- Rabies
- Rubella
- Scarlet fever
- Severe acute respiratory syndrome (SARS)
- Smallpox
- Tetanus
- Tuberculosis (TB)
- Typhus
- Viral haemorrhagic fever (VHF)
- Whooping cough
- Yellow fever

References

References to support all aspects of testing and management guidance can be found, broken up by section, by scanning the QR code below or clicking on the Resources tab on the page for this book at www.scionpublishing.com/lab_results

PART II

REQUESTING INVESTIGATIONS

The two chapters that form this part of the book aim to provide a quick reference guide to requesting appropriate investigations

- in specific clinical scenarios (*Chapter 5*)
- when patients present with various signs and/or symptoms (*Chapter 6*).

Request according to clinical judgement and local lab / referral pathway protocols – not all the tests listed will be required in all patients, and the lists are not exhaustive.

Chapter 5

Clinical scenarios

Abnormal LFT (liver screen)

Initial

- Hepatitis B and C
- Liver autoantibodies (antimitochondrial antibody, anti-smooth muscle antibody, antinuclear antibody)
- Immunoglobulins
- Ferritin and transferrin saturation (iron studies)
- USS liver

Consider

- FBC
- Coagulation
- U&E
- TFT
- HbA1c, lipids
- Coeliac screen
- Acute hepatitis: hep A, hep E, CMV, EBV
- HIV
- CK
- Serum caeruloplasmin (checking for Wilson's disease if age <40)
- Alpha-1-antitrypsin deficiency (if there is a positive FHx or associated respiratory symptoms)
- Fibrosis risk assessment if non-alcoholic fatty liver disease (NAFLD) confirmed on USS (check local protocols)

Anaemia

Initial

- FBC
- Reticulocytes
- Ferritin, iron studies
- B12, folate
- CRP
- U&E, LFT

Consider

- TFT
- Coeliac screen
- Myeloma screen
- LDH (haemolysis)
- Intrinsic factor antibodies (low B12, if not had previously and no known GI surgery that could cause malabsorption)

- Autoimmune screen, e.g. ANA, anti-CCP / RF (as per local guidance)
- Testosterone
- Haemoglobin electrophoresis (if microcytic anaemia, normal ferritin levels and not previously checked)
- Urine dipstick (haematuria)
- Stool parasites (if relevant travel history and/or eosinophilia)
- FIT: offer to all with IDA, or age ≥60 and non-IDA (colorectal cancer)
- Liver USS (liver disease)
- Pelvis USS: women age ≥55 with anaemia and visible haematuria (endometrial cancer)
- Routine OGD: age ≥55 with anaemia and upper abdominal pain (oesophageal or stomach cancer)

See also Pernicious anaemia

Antiphospholipid syndrome

Antiphospholipid syndrome is diagnosed in a patient with venous and/or arterial thrombosis and/or defined pregnancy morbidity who has persistent antiphospholipid antibodies.

- **Not** a primary care diagnosis: secondary care will likely initiate specialist review when seeing patients with thrombotic complications
- Seek specialist review if suspected, e.g.
  - VTE in the absence of major provoking factors
  - arterial thrombosis in patients aged <50 without clear risk factors
  - history of SLE or other autoimmune disease developing thrombosis or pregnancy complications
  - recurrent miscarriage (>3)

Cardiovascular disease: PAD, angina, MI, stroke

Initial

- FBC
- U&E, LFT
- HbA1c, lipids

Coeliac disease

Initial

- Coeliac serology:
  - 1st-line: total IgA and IgA tissue transglutaminase (tTG)
  - 2nd-line: IgA endomysial antibodies (EMA) if IgA tTGA testing is unavailable or IgA tTG is weakly positive
  - if IgA deficient (total IgA <0.07 g/L): IgG EMA, IgG deamidated gliadin peptide (DGP) or IgG tTG can be checked

Consider

- FBC, ferritin/iron studies, folate, B12
- TFT
- LFT, bone profile
- Vitamin D
- Repeat coeliac serology: assess adherence to a gluten-free diet

Connective tissue disease (CTD)

The 'classic' CTDs include systemic lupus erythematosus (SLE), rheumatoid arthritis (RA), systemic sclerosis (or scleroderma), polymyositis and dermatomyositis. They are often associated with certain autoantibodies, but testing should only be requested in the appropriate clinical context: they can be positive in normal individuals and are not specific for one condition. Negative results should not restrict onward referral if there are concerning clinical features.

Initial

- FBC
- ESR/CRP
- U&E, LFT
- CK
- Autoimmune screen, e.g. ANA, anti-CCP / RF (as per local guidance)
- Urine dipstick: blood ± protein present
- X ray hands and feet

Dementia

Initial

- FBC
- Ferritin/iron studies, folate, B12
- U&E, LFT, bone profile
- HbA1c
- TFT
- ESR/CRP
- Urine dipstick

Consider

- HIV
- CXR
- MRI/CT brain (as per local protocols)

Diabetes: type 1

Initial

- Assessing new-onset type 1 diabetes or diabetic ketoacidosis (DKA): point of care fingerprick blood glucose + ketones (urine or blood)

Consider (when stable)

- HbA1c
- Lipids
- U&E, LFT
- FBC
- B12, folate
- Urine ACR
- 9am cortisol
- Coeliac screen

Diabetes: type 2

Initial

- HbA1c
- FBC
- U&E, LFT
- Lipids
- Urine ACR

Consider

- Ferritin/iron studies, B12 (anaemia)

Erectile dysfunction

Initial

- HbA1c
- Lipids
- Testosterone (9–11am fasting)
- U&E, LFT

Consider

- If testosterone level is low or borderline, arrange a repeat testosterone with FSH, LH, SHBG, prolactin
- PSA
- TFT

Fibromyalgia

Fibromyalgia is a clinical diagnosis with no diagnostic specific tests.

Consider

- FBC
- ESR/CRP
- U&E, LFT, bone profile
- TFT
- CK
- HbA1C
- Autoimmune screen, e.g. ANA, anti-CCP / RF (as per local guidance)

Fungal nail infection

Initial

- Nail clippings ± scrapings for fungal MCS

Consider

- HbA1c
- FBC, U&E, LFT

Giant cell arteritis (GCA)

If suspected do not delay treatment/referral while waiting for results – seek specialist advice if needed.

Initial

- FBC
- ESR/CRP

Consider

- U&E, LFT, bone profile
- HbA1c
- Myeloma screen
- Screening tests for risk of serious infection, e.g. urine dipstick, CXR
- Screening tests for osteoporosis risk, e.g. TFT, vitamin D, DEXA

Gilbert's syndrome

Initial

- LFT
- Conjugated (direct) and unconjugated (indirect) bilirubin levels
- Clotting screen
- FBC, blood film
- Reticulocytes
- LDH

Glandular fever

Initial

- FBC and WCC differential
- Monospot or EBV serology (see *Section 4.2.2* – glandular fever re appropriate test and timings)
- LFT

Gout

Initial

- Uric acid (if <360 µmol/L but gout is strongly suspected, check level 2–4 weeks after the flare has settled)

Consider

- U&E, LFT
- Urine ACR
- Lipids, HbA1c
- Uric acid monitoring for titration of urate-lowering therapies
- X-ray symptomatic joints (erosions in established disease)

H. pylori testing

Initial

Choose one of:
- Urea (13C) breath test
- Stool Helicobacter antigen test (SAT)
- Laboratory-based serology (where locally validated)

For re-testing

- Use urea (13C) breath test

Haematuria

Initial

- FBC
- U&E
- LFT
- Urine dipstick and MCS

Consider

- PSA
- Urine ACR
- HbA1c

Haemochromatosis

Initial

- FBC
- Fasting iron studies
- U&E, LFT
- HbA1c, lipids
- *HFE* genotyping (test if a positive FHx or ↑ ferritin and ↑ transferrin saturation)

Haemolytic anaemia

Initial

- FBC
- Blood film
- Reticulocytes
- LFT
- LDH
- Urinalysis

Heart failure

Initial

- NT-pro-BNP
- FBC
- Ferritin/iron studies
- U&E, LFT
- Urine ACR

Consider

- TFT
- HbA1c
- Lipids
- Urine dipstick
- CXR

Hyper-/hypoparathyroidism

Initial

- PTH
- Bone profile
- Magnesium
- U&E
- Vitamin D

Hyperlipidaemia

Initial

- U&E, LFT
- Lipids
- HbA1c

Consider

- CK
- TFT

Hypertension

Initial

- FBC
- U&E
- LFT
- HbA1c
- Lipids
- Urine dipstick (haematuria)
- Urine ACR

Consider

- TFT

Hyperthyroidism

Initial

- TFT
- ESR/CRP: suspected thyroiditis
- FBC, LFT: if antithyroid drugs are to be started

Consider

- USS neck (palpable thyroid enlargement or focal nodularity)

Hypoadrenalism

NB: admit if clinically unwell.

Initial

- 9am cortisol
- U&E
- Glucose

Consider

- FBC
- Bone profile, LFT
- TFT

Hypopituitarism (female)

Initial (9am test)

- U&E
- FSH, LH
- Oestradiol
- Prolactin
- TFT
- Cortisol

Hypopituitarism (male)

Initial (9am test)

- U&E
- FSH, LH
- Testosterone
- Prolactin
- TFT
- Cortisol

Hypothyroidism

Initial

- TFT

Consider

- FBC, B12
- HbA1c
- Coeliac screen
- Lipids
- TPO antibodies
- USS neck (palpable thyroid enlargement or focal nodularity)

Infertility (female)

Initial

- Mid-luteal progesterone
  - if irregular bleeding, consider weekly progesterone measurements until period
- LH, FSH, prolactin, testosterone
- TFT
- Rubella status
- Chlamydia screen

Infertility (male)

Initial

- Semen analysis

Inflammatory bowel disease (IBD)

Initial

- FBC
- ESR/CRP
- U&E, LFT
- Ferritin/iron studies, B12, folate
- Vitamin D
- Coeliac screen
- TFT
- Stool MCS, including *C. difficile* toxin
- Faecal calprotectin

Irritable bowel syndrome (IBS)

Initial

- FBC
- ESR/CRP
- Coeliac screen
- Faecal calprotectin

Consider

- CA125
- Stool MCS, including *C. difficile* toxin
- FIT

Isolated raised alkaline phosphatase (ALP)

Initial

- AST/ALT, LFT
- GGT

Consider

- Bone profile, vitamin D
- Liver screen

Menopause

- Diagnose the following without FSH testing:
  - perimenopause: if vasomotor symptoms and irregular periods
  - menopause: if no period for at least 12 months (and is not using hormonal contraception)
  - menopause: based on symptoms if does not have a uterus
- Consider testing FSH to diagnose menopause in a woman, provided she is not taking combined hormonal contraception or HRT, and she is:
  - aged >45 with atypical symptoms
  - aged 40–45 with menopausal symptoms, including a change in menstrual cycle
  - aged <40 with a suspected diagnosis of premature ovarian insufficiency (POI): diagnosed with two elevated FSH levels >30IU/L taken 4–6 weeks apart
  - aged >50 using progestogen-only contraception, including depot medroxyprogesterone acetate (DMPA)
- NB: the College of Sexual and Reproductive Healthcare (CoSRH) (formerly the Faculty of Sexual and Reproductive Healthcare prior to August 2025) states that a single elevated serum FSH level (>30IU/L) indicates a degree of ovarian insufficiency, but not necessarily sterility. The British Menopause Society (BMS) recommends checking for an elevated FSH level on two blood samples taken 4–6 weeks apart

Myeloma

Initial

- FBC, blood film
- Bone profile
- U&E, LFT
- ESR/PV
- Protein electrophoresis
- Immunoglobulins
- Serum free light chains (or urine Bence Jones protein if not available)

Consider

- X-ray symptomatic areas for people with bone pain (pathological fractures)

Osteomalacia

Initial

- Vitamin D
- Bone profile
- U&E

Consider

- PTH
- FBC
- Ferritin/iron studies, folate B12
- LFT
- TFT
- Coeliac screen

Osteoporosis

Initial

- FBC
- ESR/CRP
- U&E, LFT, bone profile
- Vitamin D
- FRAX score (assess need for DEXA)

Consider tests for secondary causes

- Female with irregular periods: oestradiol, FSH, LH, prolactin
- Male with suspected hypogonadism: testosterone, FSH, LH, SHBG, prolactin
- Diabetes: HbA1c, lipids
- Hyperthyroidism: TFT
- Hyperparathyroidism: PTH
- Rheumatological: autoimmune screen, e.g. ANA, anti-CCP / RF (as per local guidance)
- Coeliac screen
- Myeloma screen

Pancytopenia

This is a decrease in all three haematological cell lines (red cells, white cells and platelets) with many causes. If unwell or severe features (e.g. Hb <8, platelets <20, WCC <0.5, abnormal blood film), likely to need emergency admission.

Initial

- FBC, blood film
- Coagulation
- ESR/CRP
- Reticulocytes
- B12, folate
- U&E, LFT, bone profile
- Coeliac screen

Consider

- Myeloma screen
- Autoimmune screen, e.g. ANA, anti-CCP / RF (as per local guidance)
- Viral screen (e.g. EBV, CMV, HIV, hepatitis B and C)

Pernicious anaemia

Initial

- FBC
- Ferritin/iron studies, folate, B12
- Coeliac screen
- Intrinsic factor antibody

Polycystic ovarian syndrome (PCOS)

Initial

- Total testosterone, SHBG, FAI
- FSH, LH
- Prolactin
- TFT

Consider

- USS pelvis (unless the diagnosis is obvious on clinical and biochemical grounds)
- HbA1c
- Lipids

Polymyalgia rheumatica (PMR)

Initial

- FBC
- ESR/CRP
- U&E, LFT
- Bone profile, vitamin D
- TFT
- CK
- Autoimmune screen, e.g. ANA, anti-CCP / RF (as per local guidance)

Consider

- Myeloma screen
- CXR

Primary immunodeficiency

The diagnosis cannot be excluded based on normal blood tests alone. Perform tests when there are no symptoms of infection.

Initial

- FBC
- Immunoglobulins
- U&E, LFT
- HIV

Restless legs syndrome

There are no investigations to confirm the diagnosis.

Initial

- Ferritin

Consider

- FBC
- Folate, B12
- U&E, LFT
- TFT
- HbA1c

Sickle cell disease

The choice of test will depend on local guidelines and facilities: seek advice about the appropriate tests.

Initial

- FBC, blood film
- Reticulocytes
- Hb electrophoresis

Spondyloarthritis

Spondyloarthritis is a term describing a group of clinically heterogeneous inflammatory rheumatologic conditions. It may be predominantly axial, affecting the sacroiliac joints and the spine, or predominantly peripheral (commonly psoriatic arthritis). It cannot be reliably diagnosed or ruled out by a single test. Do not let investigations delay a referral for clinically suspected spondyloarthritis or psoriatic arthropathy.

Initial

- FBC
- ESR/CRP
- U&E, LFT
- Bone profile, vitamin D
- Uric acid
- TFT
- Autoimmune screen, e.g. ANA, anti-CCP / RF (as per local guidance)

- HLA-B27: if age <45 and low back pain >3 months and three of the following to decide if rheumatology referral needed (refer if positive):
  - low back pain starting before age 35
  - symptoms which wake them during the second half of the night
  - buttock pain
  - improvement when moving
  - improvement within 48 hours of taking an NSAID
  - spondyloarthritis in a 1st-degree relative
  - current or past arthritis
  - current or past enthesitis
  - current or past psoriasis

Consider

- Plain film X-rays (check local protocol) of the:
  - sacroiliac joints and spine: in suspected axial spondyloarthritis to identify sacroiliitis, sclerosis (thickening of bone), erosions, and partial or total ankylosis (fusion of joints)
  - hands and feet: in suspected psoriatic arthritis to identify erosion in the distal interphalangeal joint and periarticular new bone formation. Soft tissue swelling may be the only radiographic finding in early disease
  - pelvis: in all people with suspected psoriatic arthritis, as there is a high rate of asymptomatic damage
- Ultrasound of the joints of hands and feet and suspected enthesitis sites (check local protocol): in suspected psoriatic arthropathy if a diagnosis cannot be made from a plain film X-ray

Suspected cancer

Initial

- FBC
- ESR/CRP
- Ferritin, iron studies, B12, folate
- U&E, LFT, bone profile

Consider

- PSA
- CA125, USS pelvis
- HbA1c
- Myeloma screen
- Urine dipstick
- FIT
- CXR

Thalassaemia

Initial

- FBC
- Blood film
- Reticulocytes
- Hb electrophoresis
- LFT

Thrombophilia

In primary care, it is best to refer to haematology to guide the appropriateness of testing. Results may not affect management and testing is often not exhaustive, i.e. negative tests do not rule out an inherited thrombotic tendency.

Vasculitis

These are a varied group of rare diseases characterised by inflammation of blood vessels. They are difficult to diagnose because the clinical manifestations are varied and can mimic several infectious, neoplastic, and other autoimmune conditions. Refer to a specialist for definitive diagnosis.

Consider

- FBC
- U&E, LFT
- ESR/CRP
- Urine dipstick

References

References to support all aspects of testing and management guidance can be found, broken up by section, by scanning the QR code below or clicking on the Resources tab on the page for this book at www.scionpublishing.com/lab_results

Signs and symptoms

Follow your local reference ranges, clinical pathways, management and referral guidance. This guidance is not a substitute for individual clinical judgement. Reference ranges will vary according to the assay used by laboratories. Those provided are examples and may vary in your locality.

Abdominal pain

Initial

- FBC
- CRP
- U&E, LFT, bone profile
- HbA1c/glucose

Consider

- CA125
- PSA
- Urine pregnancy test
- Urine dipstick ± MCS
- STI screen
- Stool MCS
- FIT
- Faecal calprotectin
- *H. pylori* testing

Acute confusion (delirium)

Consider

- FBC
- ESR, CRP
- Folate, B12
- U&E, LFT, bone profile
- TFT
- HbA1c/glucose
- Urine dipstick ± MCS

Allergy

This is primarily a clinical diagnosis: tests are used to help confirm or refute a diagnosis. Follow appropriate local testing and referral procedures. Note, there are no tests for food intolerance.

Consider

- Specific IgE testing: to support clinical diagnosis in suspected IgE-mediated allergies
- Check total IgE when testing specific IgE

Alopecia

Consider

- FBC
- Ferritin
- TFT
- Skin scrapings and hair samples for fungal MCS

Altered bowel habit

Initial

- FBC
- U&E, LFT, bone profile
- ESR/CRP
- Coeliac screen

Consider

- TFT
- CA125
- Faecal calprotectin
- Stool MCS, including *C. difficile* toxin
- FIT

Amenorrhoea (primary)

Initial (likely to be investigated by secondary care)

- Urine pregnancy test
- Prolactin
- TFT
- FSH, LH
- Oestradiol
- Total testosterone
- Coeliac screen
- USS pelvis

Amenorrhoea (secondary)

Initial

- Urine pregnancy test
- Prolactin
- TFT

- FSH, LH
- Oestradiol
- Total testosterone
- USS pelvis (suspected PCOS, unless the diagnosis is obvious on clinical and biochemical grounds)

Angular cheilitis

Initial

- FBC
- Folate, B12, ferritin/iron studies
- Skin swab for MCS, viral swab

Ankle swelling

Initial

- NT-pro-BNP
- FBC
- Ferritin/iron studies
- U&E, LFT
- Urine ACR

Consider

- TFT
- HbA1c
- Lipids
- Urine dipstick
- CXR

Back pain

Consider

- FBC
- ESR/CRP
- U&E, LFT
- Bone profile, vitamin D
- PSA
- CA125
- Autoimmune screen, e.g. ANA, anti-CCP / RF (as per local guidance)
- HLA-B27 (see spondyloarthritis section in *Chapter 5*)
- Myeloma screen (persistent back pain, age ≥60)
- HIV
- Urine dipstick

- FIT
- CXR
- Direct access CT, or USS if not available for pancreatic cancer (back pain with weight loss, age ≥60)
- Spinal X-ray: if there is suspicion of a specific pathology, e.g. compression fracture due to osteoporosis or bone pain due to malignancy

Chest pain

NB: Troponins should not be requested in primary care.

Initial

- HbA1c, lipids
- FBC
- U&E, LFT
- TFT
- ESR/CRP
- CXR

Clubbing

Initial

- FBC
- U&E, LFT, bone profile
- ESR/CRP

Consider

- Lung causes: sputum MCS, CXR
- Cancer: suspected cancer screen (see *Suspected cancer* in *Chapter 5*)
- GI: liver screen, faecal calprotectin, coeliac screen, stool for parasites
- Endocrine: TFT
- Infection: HIV

Constipation

Consider

- FBC
- Ferritin/iron studies, folate, B12
- ESR/CRP
- HbA1c
- Bone profile, PTH, magnesium, U&E
- TFT

Cough

Initial

- FBC
- ESR/CRP
- Sputum MCS
- CXR

Diarrhoea, acute (<4 weeks)

Initial

- Stool MCS if:
  - there are symptoms/signs or a clinical indication:
    - systemically unwell; needs hospital admission and/or antibiotics
    - blood or pus in the stool
    - immunocompromised
    - recently received antibiotics, a PPI or been in hospital (also request specific testing for *C. difficile*)
    - foreign travel: request tests for ova, cysts, and parasites and state the countries visited
    - amoebae, *Giardia*, or cryptosporidium are suspected: if diarrhoea is persistent (2 weeks or more) or the person has travelled to an at-risk area
    - need to exclude infectious diarrhoea, e.g. severe abdominal pain, exacerbation of IBD or IBS
  - there is a public health indication:
    - diarrhoea in high-risk people, e.g. food handlers, healthcare workers, elderly residents in care homes
    - suspected food poisoning, e.g. after a barbecue or restaurant meal or eating eggs, chicken or shellfish
    - outbreaks of diarrhoea in the family or community, when isolating the organism, may help pinpoint the source of the outbreak
    - contacts of people infected with certain organisms, e.g. *Escherichia coli* O157 or *C. difficile*, where there may be serious clinical sequelae to an infection
    - close household contacts of a person with a *Giardia* infection
- Blood tests if infection has been excluded and it is suspected that an episode of acute diarrhoea is due to a chronic cause (*see* Diarrhoea, chronic (>4 weeks))

Diarrhoea, chronic (>4 weeks)

Initial

- FBC
- U&E, LFT, bone profile
- B12, folate

- Ferritin/iron studies
- TFT
- ESR/CRP
- Coeliac screen

Consider

- CA125
- HIV
- Stool for:
  - routine microbiology investigation and examination for ova, cysts and parasites (travel history)
    - send three specimens at least 2 days apart, as ova, cysts and parasites are shed intermittently
  - *C. difficile* testing (recent hospital admission or antibiotics/PPI, previous episode)
  - faecal calprotectin (differentiate between IBS and IBD in those aged <40 if specialist assessment is being considered and cancer is not suspected)
  - FIT (symptoms suggestive of colorectal cancer who do not meet suspected cancer referral pathway criteria)

Dizziness and syncope

Initial

- FBC
- Glucose, HbA1c
- U&E, LFT
- Urine pregnancy test
- CXR

Dyspareunia

Consider

- CA125
- Urine dipstick
- Vaginal swabs for MCS
- STI screen
- USS pelvis

Dysphagia

Initial

- FBC
- ESR/CRP
- U&E, LFT, bone profile

- Ferritin/iron studies
- OGD: offer urgent, direct access upper GI endoscopy (to be done within 2 weeks, oesophageal or stomach cancer)

Easy bruising

This is common, but a primary haematological cause is rarely found. With new sudden onset bruising, consider urgent FBC and coagulation screen to exclude acute leukaemia, especially if associated with weight loss, fever, hepatosplenomegaly. NB: an abnormal screen does not necessarily indicate an increase in the risk of bleeding; a normal screen does not rule out a bleeding disorder.

Initial

- FBC, blood film
- Coagulation
- U&E, LFT, TFT
- Urine dipstick

Excess sweating

Initial

- FBC, blood film
- ESR/CRP
- U&E, LFT
- HbA1c
- TFT
- HIV
- CXR

Galactorrhoea

Initial

- Prolactin

Consider

- TFT
- U&E
- Urine pregnancy test
- Hypogonadism screen: oestradiol or testosterone, LH, FSH

Gynaecomastia

Initial

- U&E, LFT
- TFT

Consider

- Testosterone, SHBG
- LH, FSH
- Oestrogen
- Prolactin

Haematospermia

Initial

- Urine dipstick and MCS
- PSA
- U&E, LFT

Consider

- FBC
- Coagulation
- Semen MCS if infection is suspected, e.g. TB, schistosomiasis
- USS scrotum

Haemoptysis

NB: follow local pathways for D-dimer requests (may be secondary care only).

Initial

- FBC
- Coagulation
- ESR/CRP
- U&E, LFT
- CXR

Consider

- Sputum MCS

Heavy menstrual bleeding

Initial

- FBC

Consider

- Ferritin/iron studies
- TFT
- Coagulation
- Urine pregnancy test
- STI screen

Hepatomegaly

Initial

- FBC, blood film
- U&E, LFT
- Coagulation
- ESR/CRP
- Liver screen
- USS liver (urgent)

Hirsutism

Initial

- Testosterone, SHBG, free androgen index (FAI)
- TFT
- Prolactin
- FSH, LH

Incontinence (female)

Initial

- Urine dipstick
- U&E
- HbA1c

Consider

- CA125

Indigestion

Initial

- FBC
- ESR/CRP
- Coeliac screen
- U&E, LFT
- Ferritin/iron studies

Consider

- *H. pylori* testing
- Stool MCS
- Faecal calprotectin
- Direct access OGD (oesophageal or stomach cancer)
  - aged ≥55 with weight loss and any of the following: upper abdominal pain, reflux, dyspepsia (urgent)
  - aged ≥55 with any of the following (consider non-urgent):
    - **dyspepsia** (treatment-resistant)
    - **dyspepsia** with raised platelet count or nausea or vomiting
    - **haemoglobin levels low** with upper abdominal pain
    - **nausea or vomiting** with raised platelet count or weight loss or reflux or dyspepsia or upper abdominal pain
    - **platelet count raised** with nausea or vomiting or weight loss or reflux or dyspepsia or upper abdominal pain
    - **reflux** with raised platelet count or nausea or vomiting
    - **upper abdominal pain** with low haemoglobin levels or raised platelet count or nausea or vomiting
    - **weight loss** with raised platelet count or nausea or vomiting

Inflammatory arthritis

Refer if strong clinical suspicion, even if tests are normal.

Initial

- FBC
- ESR/CRP
- U&E, LFT
- Autoimmune screen, e.g. ANA, anti-CCP / RF (as per local guidance)
- Urine dipstick: blood ± protein present
- X-rays hands and feet: can be normal in early disease; soft tissue changes (swelling, effusions, calcification); bony changes (more advanced disease)

Jaundice

Initial

- FBC
- U&E, LFT
- Coagulation
- Hepatitis B and C
- Liver screen
- Urine dipstick
- USS abdomen

Leg ulcers

Initial

- FBC
- ESR/CRP
- U&E, LFT
- HbA1c
- Wound swabs for MCS if suspicion of infection

Loss of appetite

Initial

- FBC
- Ferritin/iron studies
- U&E, LFT, bone profile

Consider

- TFT
- PSA
- CA125
- FIT
- Urine dipstick
- CXR

Low libido (female)

Initial

- FBC
- HbA1c
- U&E, LFT
- TFT

- Consider secondary amenorrhoea investigations if relevant (see *Amenorrhoea (secondary)* earlier in this chapter)

Low libido (male)

Initial

- Testosterone, SHBG
- FSH, LH
- Prolactin
- FBC

Lower urinary tract symptoms (LUTS) – male

Initial

- Urine dipstick
- U&E

Consider

- PSA

Lymphadenopathy

Initial

- FBC, blood film, ESR/CRP
- U&E, LFT, bone profile

Consider

- Myeloma screen
- Glandular fever screen
- HIV
- Autoimmune screen, e.g. ANA, anti-CCP / RF (as per local guidance)
- PSA
- CA125
- Relevant imaging, e.g. CXR (for people aged ≥40 with supraclavicular lymphadenopathy or persistent cervical lymphadenopathy)
- USS assessment (if mild lymphadenopathy and no concerning features)

Mouth ulcers

Consider

- FBC
- ESR/CRP

- Ferritin/iron studies, folate, B12
- Coeliac screen
- HIV
- Glandular fever screen
- Autoimmune screen, e.g. ANA
- Faecal calprotectin

Nausea and vomiting

Consider

- FBC
- ESR/CRP
- U&E, LFT, bone profile
- Urine pregnancy test
- *H. pylori* testing
- Stool MCS
- HbA1c
- TFT
- 9am cortisol
- Relevant imaging, e.g. CXR, USS abdomen/pelvis

Night sweats

Initial

- FBC, blood film
- ESR/CRP
- U&E, LFT, bone profile
- HbA1c
- TFT

Consider

- Myeloma screen
- Glandular fever screen
- HIV
- Autoimmune screen, e.g. ANA, anti-CCP / RF (as per local guidance)
- FSH for menopause if appropriate
- Relevant imaging, e.g. CXR

Obesity

Consider

- HbA1c, lipids
- TFT
- U&E, LFT

Paget's disease

Initial

- Plain X-ray of affected area
- Bone profile, LFT, U&E, vitamin D

Painful muscles

Consider

- CK
- FBC
- ESR/CRP
- U&E, LFT
- TFT
- Autoimmune screen, e.g. ANA, anti-CCP / RF (as per local guidance)

Painful tongue (glossitis)

Consider

- FBC
- Ferritin/iron studies, folate, B12
- Coeliac screen

Palpitations

Consider

- FBC
- U&E, LFT
- TFT
- HbA1c/glucose

Pelvic pain (female)

Consider

- Urine dipstick, MCS
- Urine pregnancy test
- Vaginal swabs for MCS
- Sexually transmitted infection (STI) screen
- CA125
- USS pelvis

Penile discharge

Consider

- Penile swabs for MCS
- STI screen
- HbA1c
- HIV, hepatitis B and C
- Urine dipstick

Peripheral neuropathy

Initial

- FBC
- ESR/CRP
- HbA1c, lipids
- TFT
- B12, folate

Consider

- Myeloma screen
- HIV, hepatitis B and C
- Autoimmune screen, e.g. ANA, anti-CCP / RF (as per local guidance)

Polydipsia

Initial

- Glucose, HbA1c
- Bone profile
- U&E
- Urine dipstick

Consider

- Urine and plasma osmolality

Pruritus (generalised)

Consider

- FBC
- Ferritin/iron studies
- U&E, LFT
- TFT

- HbA1c
- Bone profile
- HIV, hepatitis B and C
- Relevant imaging, e.g. CXR, USS abdomen

Raynaud's phenomenon

Initial

- FBC
- ESR/CRP
- U&E, LFT
- TFT
- Autoimmune screen, e.g. ANA, anti-CCP / RF (as per local guidance)

Rectal bleeding

Initial

- FBC
- Ferritin/iron studies
- ESR/CRP
- U&E, LFT, bone profile

Consider

- FIT
- Faecal calprotectin
- Stool MCS

Shortness of breath

NB: follow local pathways for D-dimer requests (may be secondary care only).

Initial

- FBC
- Coagulation
- ESR/CRP
- U&E, LFT
- CXR

Consider

- Sputum MCS
- NT-pro-BNP
- TFT

Single joint pain

Initial

- FBC
- ESR/CRP
- U&E, LFT
- Urate
- X-ray symptomatic joints

Sore throat

Consider

- Throat swab for MCS
- Glandular fever screen
- HIV
- Urgent FBC if taking relevant medications, e.g. disease-modifying antirheumatic drugs (DMARDs), carbimazole

Splenomegaly

Initial

- FBC, blood film
- ESR/CRP
- U&E, LFT, bone profile

Consider

- Myeloma screen
- Glandular fever screen
- Viral screen, e.g. EBV, CMV, HIV, hepatitis B and C
- Autoimmune screen, e.g. ANA, anti-CCP / RF (as per local guidance)
- USS abdomen
- Haemolysis screen (blood film, reticulocyte count, LDH, bilirubin)

Steatorrhoea

Consider

- FBC
- ESR/CRP
- Coeliac screen
- U&E, LFT
- TFT
- HIV

- Faecal elastase
- Stool MCS, stool for ova, cysts and parasites
- Faecal calprotectin

Tinnitus

Consider

- FBC
- U&E
- HbA1c, lipids
- TFT

Tired all the time (TATT)

Initial

- FBC, blood film
- Ferritin/iron studies, folate, B12, vitamin D
- ESR/CRP
- U&E, LFT, bone profile
- HbA1c
- TFT
- Coeliac screen
- Urine dipstick

Consider

- NT-pro-BNP
- 9am cortisol
- Myeloma screen
- Glandular fever screen
- Hypopituitarism screen
- CK
- HIV, hepatitis B and C
- CA125
- PSA
- Autoimmune screen, e.g. ANA, anti-CCP / RF (as per local guidance)
- Relevant imaging, e.g. CXR

Tremor

Consider

- U&E, LFT, bone profile
- TFT

Unexplained weight gain

Consider

- FBC
- U&E, LFT
- HbA1c, lipids
- TFT
- CA125
- PCOS investigation
- Urine dipstick
- Urine pregnancy test
- USS abdomen/pelvis

Unexplained weight loss

Initial

- FBC
- ESR/CRP
- Ferritin, iron studies, B12, folate
- U&E, LFT, bone profile

Consider

- TFT
- HbA1c
- Myeloma screen
- PSA
- CA125, USS pelvis
- HIV
- Urine dipstick
- FIT
- CXR

Urinary tract infection (female)

Consider

- FBC
- ESR/CRP
- U&E, bone profile
- Urine dipstick, urine MCS
- CA125
- HbA1c
- Urine pregnancy test
- Vaginal swabs for MCS, STI screen

Urinary tract infection (male)

Initial

- Urine MCS

Consider

- Urine dipstick
- FBC
- ESR/CRP
- U&E, bone profile
- HbA1c
- STI screen

Urticaria

Consider

- FBC
- LFT
- TFT
- ESR/CRP
- *H. pylori* testing
- Hepatitis B and C
- Urine dipstick

Vaginal discharge

Consider

- High vaginal swabs for MCS
- STI screen
- Urine pregnancy test
- Urine dipstick

References

References to support all aspects of testing and management guidance can be found, broken up by section, by scanning the QR code below or clicking on the Resources tab on the page for this book at www.scionpublishing.com/lab_results

Index